The Million-Dollar Misdiagnosis

The Million-Dollar Misdiagnosis

Suzanne H Visser

CONTENTS

For all people living with Bertolotti Syndrome.

For those still searching for a name for their pain; for those who have been dismissed, doubted, misdiagnosed or told that nothing serious is wrong; for those who have spent years trying to explain a body that others have not properly seen; and for those who continue to build lives of courage, humour, work, care and creativity around a condition that asks far too much.

PROLOGUE

Most people think of a life in years, jobs, houses, relationships and achievements. I have learned to think of mine in smaller units. Fifteen minutes at the sink. Fifteen minutes at the stove. Fifteen minutes standing before my body begins to insist on the horizontal. Fifteen minutes sorting papers, folding clothes, chopping vegetables, putting paintings away, packing books, answering messages, or doing some other ordinary tasks that most people would not think of as physical labour.

For me, ordinary life has become physical labour.

This is not because I am frail by temperament. It is not because I have failed to try hard enough, stretch enough, meditate enough, exercise enough, think positively enough, forgive enough, journal enough, or drink enough green juice. I have done all of that, and more. For almost fifty years I tried to solve a problem that nobody had properly named. Doctors looked at my spine, my muscles, my posture, my emotions, my stress, my childhood, my personality and my supposed pain identity. They looked everywhere except at the small piece of abnormal anatomy that was causing the trouble.

The condition is called Bertolotti Syndrome. I was born with it. In simple terms, one of the lower vertebrae in my spine developed in an abnormal way. A bony wing at the base of the spine sits where it should not sit, moves where it should not move, and presses or grinds in ways the body was not designed to tolerate. In some people, this anatomical variation causes no pain at all. In others, it becomes a source of chronic and sometimes disabling pain. In my case, it shaped almost everything.

For most of my life, I did not know that.

I knew only that my back hurt. It hurt when I was young. It hurt after childbirth. It hurt when I lifted babies, carried shopping, stood too long, sat too long, walked too far, bent down, straightened up, travelled, worked, cooked, cleaned, wrote, danced, rested, hoped, and tried again. The pain was not always the same. Sometimes it was a deep grinding ache. Sometimes it was a sudden attack, as if a string in my back had been plucked. Sometimes it spread into fatigue so complete that the whole body seemed to lose voltage. Sometimes it made me irritable, sometimes frightened, sometimes ashamed. Mostly, it made me practical.

Practicality is underrated. Pain strips life down to logistics. Where is the chair? How long can I sit in it? Where can I lie down afterwards? How far is the car from the door? Can I carry that bag? Can I stand long enough to cook this meal? Can I make it through coffee with a friend? Can I attend the appointment and still work later? Can I survive the scan, the waiting room, the hard chair, the bright lights, the cheerful dismissal?

Because I could not trust my body, I had to become a manager of time, movement and consequence. I learned to calculate the cost of every action. I learned that a full dishwasher was not merely a full dishwasher. It was bending, lifting, twisting, reaching, unloading, standing, and paying later. I learned that a saucepan could be too heavy, that a floor could be too far away, that a shower could be an event, that packing a suitcase could require strategy, and that standing at a sink could become one of the hardest tasks in the house.

I also learned that a life can still be made.

This book is about pain, but it is not a book in which pain gets the whole stage. Pain has already taken enough. This is also a book about writing, painting, publishing, cooking, legal scholarship, friendship, humour, stubbornness, style, work, thought and the strange discipline of building a life from fragments. It is about the books I wrote, the poems I made, the paintings I gave away, the meals I cooked, the publishing house

I founded, the legal ideas I followed, and the PhD thesis I completed while lying down. It is about the fact that a body can become smaller in its range while a life remains intellectually and creatively large.

For years, I thought my problem was that I needed to fix myself. I moved countries. I tried doctors, chiropractors, physiotherapists, acupuncturists, massage therapists, healers, spiritual teachers, supplements, diets, shoes, wedges, machines, exercises, yoga, meditation, bodywork, medication, and almost every respectable and disreputable theory about back pain that came across my path. I took the advice seriously. I tried to be a good patient. I tried to be a better person. I tried to become more relaxed, more conscious, more forgiving, more embodied, more disciplined, more psychologically honest, more spiritually evolved.

The pain remained.

By the time the correct diagnosis arrived, I had spent approximately $1.2 million (Australian dollars) trying to treat the condition without knowing what it was. That figure is approximate. It includes medical consultations, alternative treatments, equipment, special shoes, exercise regimes, medication, travel, lost opportunities, reduced earning capacity, interrupted work, and the slow economic leakage that follows a body through decades of unmanaged pain. It is not a single bill. It is the cost of not knowing. It is the price of being sent down every road except the one that led to the actual problem.

The money matters, but it is not the greatest loss. The greater loss is time. Time spent explaining yourself to people who are not listening. Time spent trying to prove that the pain is real. Time spent doing exercises for the wrong condition. Time spent apologising for limitations you do not yet understand. Time spent wondering whether the problem might, after all, be your fault.

When I finally heard the words Bertolotti Syndrome, the diagnosis did not cure me. It did something else. It ended the madness. It closed the gap between what I felt in my body and what I had been told to believe. The pain was not a moral failure. It was not repressed anger. It was not a lack of mindfulness. It was not a stubborn attachment to suffering. It was anatomy.

There is relief in that. There is grief as well.

A diagnosis late in life is a strange gift. It gives meaning to what has already been lost. It rearranges the past without returning it. The child who stumbled over her own feet, the young mother with the wrong shoes, the dancer with one impossible side, the woman in Japan trying to understand the violent messages from her back, the patient in Australia being told yet again that nothing serious could be seen, the writer lying down with a computer balanced into the least painful position: all of them suddenly belong to the same story.

This book is that story.

It begins with a body that was speaking before anyone knew how to listen. It moves through childhood, dance, childbirth, misdiagnosis, alternative medicine, Japan, Australia, law, publishing, art, cooking, friendship, housing stress, and the stubborn practice of keeping a life going. It returns often to the Dutch saying commonly associated with the famous soccer player Johan Cruijff: every disadvantage has its advantage. I have always liked that sentence because it is not sentimental. It does not say that suffering is good. It does not say that pain ennobles. It says something more interesting and more exact: disadvantage may contain an advantage, provided one is ruthless enough, inventive enough or desperate enough to find it.

The advantage in my case was never Bertolotti Syndrome itself. The advantage was what the condition forced me to learn. It forced me to become exact with time. It forced me to distinguish between the essential and the decorative. It forced me to work in short, concentrated bursts. It forced me to think before moving. It forced me to make systems. It forced me to rest before collapse. It forced me to create from the horizontal.

It also forced me to see how often systems fail people by looking in the wrong place. A doctor can miss the structure that causes the pain. A legal system can miss the human being behind the category. A university can miss the actual question because it is too busy protecting its procedure. A society can miss the disabled person because she looks capable, speaks clearly, writes books, runs a business, cooks beautifully, and still manages to laugh.

Competence can hide suffering. Productivity can hide disability. Intelligence can make people assume you are coping better than you are.

I have often appeared more functional than I felt. I could write. I could speak. I could produce. I could run a publishing house. I could complete academic work. I could make paintings. I could cook. I could organise. I could still be useful. This confused people, including doctors. They seemed to think that if the mind was bright, the body could not be as bad as I said it was. They did not understand that the mind had become bright partly because the body had forced me into stillness. Study, reading, meditation, writing and art became ways of surviving without surrendering the whole self to pain.

Now I live by arrangement. I swim. I use a Pilates reformer. I rebound when I can. I lie down to work. I avoid medication as much as possible. I rest more than I want to. I use a walking stick. I drop things. My hands are affected. I invite friends for Japanese tea ceremony partly because beauty matters and partly because my hands need the practice. I see people in short bursts. Two hours in a café is my absolute maximum. Standing at the sink is nearly impossible. Ready-made meals sometimes stand between me and exhaustion.

Yet I am still here. I am still writing. I am still studying. I am still thinking. I am still making.

This is not a triumph-over-adversity story. I do not like that genre. I have not triumphed over Bertolotti Syndrome. I live with it. Some days I live with it badly. Some days I live with it efficiently. Some days I live with it with rage. Some days I live with it with tea, swimming, a poem, a manuscript, a painting, a legal idea, a good meal, or a friend who knows that I may need to lie down before the conversation is finished.

That is the truth of this book. The body has been a tyrant, but it has not been the whole government.

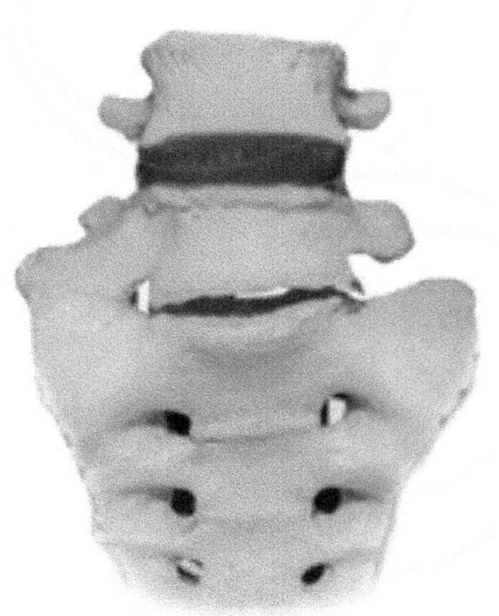

1

Ghent, 1978

The pain began properly in Belgium.

Before that, there had been signs: the stumbling child, the inward-turning foot, the one-sided body, the split I could do on one side and not the other, the strange pain in the groin that no amount of training could overcome. But signs are not the same as an adult life organised around pain. Childhood gave warnings. Belgium gave the first sentence of the life that followed.

I was twenty-one, living in Ghent with my young family, and I had just given birth to my first child. I was also a dancer. That matters because it means my body was not neglected, weak, lazy or untouched by discipline. I had spent years training it. I had done classical ballet in my teens, and although I had been rejected by a professional ballet school, I continued to dance. I studied with Min Tanaka, the Japanese dancer who gave workshops in Europe at the time. My body was strong, stretched, trained and responsive in many ways. I could do things with it that most people could not do.

I could sit with my legs spread and lower my upper body all the way to the floor. That kind of movement requires discipline, breath, repetition and trust in the body. But even there, in the middle of skill, the old asymmetry remained. From that position, I could roll one leg backwards on one side only. My fellow dancers could do it on both sides. I could not. It did not matter how much I trained. It remained impossible.

That word is important: impossible.

Dancers are used to difficulty. They are not easily impressed by discomfort. They know the difference between stiffness and refusal, between a body that needs more repetition and a body that has reached a boundary. This was not reluctance. It was not lack of effort. It was not fear. Something in the structure of my body would not allow the movement. I had no medical language for it, but I knew the difference in practice. One side belonged to dance. The other side belonged to mystery.

Then came motherhood.

My first child was a heavy baby. Carrying him was difficult. He sat on my right hip because that worked better than the left. My right hip seemed higher, or somehow more available, although that is only the language I had then. A mother with a baby does not usually conduct a biomechanical analysis of how she carries the child. She carries the child where the body permits it. She adjusts. She shifts the baby from one side to the other. She finds the position that allows her to keep going. If that position is crooked, she becomes crooked. If it costs her later, she pays later.

I went to my general practitioner because my lower back hurt. He told me that some lower back pain was normal after giving birth.

This was both plausible and useless.

Of course childbirth changes the body. Of course pregnancy and carrying a baby can strain the back. Of course a young mother may hurt. The danger of a plausible explanation is that it can stop the search too early. Once pain is placed inside a category called "normal after childbirth", the particular body disappears. The doctor no longer has to ask why this back, this hip, this pattern, this history, this one-sidedness, this pain. The general explanation swallows the specific one.

The doctor recommended the kind of mules nurses wore at the time: wooden soles with a thin anti-slip rubber layer and leather tops. Shoes as diagnosis. Shoes as treatment. Shoes as the first official attempt to turn a structural problem into a practical adjustment.

I wore them, or at least tried to. I was young, busy, in pain and willing to believe that someone knew what he was doing. That is one of the humiliations of being a patient. You are required to trust people who may be wrong. You do not yet know they are wrong. You only know they speak with authority, and you are tired.

My second child was born eleven months later.

There was no spacious recovery between the two births. There was no long interval in which the body could reorganise itself, recover strength, settle, and be studied carefully. There were now two babies. Two small bodies to lift, carry, feed, wash, comfort, move and protect. Two children in a house where the work was immediate, repetitive and physical. Two children before my own body had found its way back from the first.

I had to pick up babies all day. I had to bend and lift. I had to carry the weight of motherhood literally, not as metaphor. A baby does not wait for the mother's lower back to improve. A child does not understand that the person holding him may be negotiating with pain. Small children make urgent claims on the body. They require repetition without regard for injury.

The backache worsened.

A physiotherapist then offered a more dramatic explanation. He said my right leg was at least three centimetres shorter than my left.

Three centimetres is a large measurement inside a human body. It is large enough to organise a life around. It is large enough to explain asymmetry, or so it seemed. It gave a number to what had previously been vague. The right hip, the odd stance, the history of one-sidedness, the pain after childbirth: suddenly all of it could be placed under the heading of a short leg.

A special right shoe was made with a three-centimetre-thick sole.

I can still feel the absurd seriousness of that object. A shoe can become a form of medical authority. It says: we have measured you. We have found the problem. This is the correction. Wear it, and the body will be brought into order.

But the body did not come into order. The pain did not disappear. It became worse.

At the time, I did not have the knowledge to challenge the premise. If someone said one leg was shorter, perhaps one leg was shorter. If someone made a shoe, perhaps the shoe was necessary. If the pain grew worse, perhaps the body was still adjusting. Perhaps I had to persist. Perhaps I was not wearing it correctly. Perhaps everything took time.

A wrong diagnosis has a peculiar power. It does not merely fail to help. It recruits the patient into its logic. Once the explanation has been given, the patient begins to interpret her own suffering through it. If the special shoe hurts, the mind looks for reasons the shoe might still be right. If the treatment does not work, the patient wonders whether she has misunderstood, or failed to comply, or expected too much too quickly. A person in pain can become very obedient to nonsense when nonsense arrives wearing professional clothes.

The shoe also did something more serious. It altered the way I stood and walked. It changed the load through a body that was already compensating. It tried to correct a leg-length problem when the deeper issue was not a simple leg-length problem at all. Decades later, after the diagnosis, the old asymmetry would make a different kind of sense. But at the time, the shoe became another intervention in a body that had not been properly understood.

I was not living in a medical textbook. I was living in the chaos of small children, jobs, housekeeping and ordinary survival. That is another reason misdiagnosis lasts. Life does not pause while the body is being investigated. A young mother cannot spend her days constructing a perfect account of symptoms. She cannot stop all obligations and wait for diagnostic clarity. She carries on. The pain becomes part of the furniture of the day.

There were meals to make, children to hold, work to do, floors to clean, washing to manage, arrangements to make, money to think about, fatigue to ignore. Pain entered all of it quietly and then not quietly. It did not announce itself as a permanent life companion. It arrived first as something that should pass, then as something that had not passed, then as something that seemed to belong to me.

This is how chronic pain colonises a life. At first, one says, my back hurts. Later, one says, I have a bad back. Later still, the bad back becomes part of every decision before the decision is even made.

I did not yet know how much the pain would cost. I did not know that this was the beginning of decades of consultations, treatments, equipment, shoes, exercises, alternative therapies, scans, medication, wasted hope and wasted money. I did not know that I would eventually calculate the cost of not knowing at approximately $1.2 million. At twenty-one, with two children and a worsening back, I knew only that something was wrong and that the people I asked did not know what it was.

This is the part of the story where the reader may want someone to intervene. Someone should ask the right question. Someone should notice that the young woman was a dancer with an old history of asymmetry. Someone should connect the childhood stumbling, the inward-turning foot, the one-sided split, the groin pain, the higher hip, the back pain after childbirth and the worsening pain after the raised shoe. Someone should say: perhaps this is structural. Perhaps the pelvis and spine need to be looked at together. Perhaps the base of the spine matters.

No one did.

Instead, the pain became domesticated. It lived in the house with us. It came to the shops, the kitchen, the bedroom, the street, the dance studio, the doctor's office. It sat with me while I nursed babies. It followed me when I carried them. It stood behind me while I bent over baths, beds, prams, bags and washing. It became part of motherhood without being named.

That matters because motherhood already asks the body to disappear. The baby's needs come first, then the older child's, then the household's, then the job's, then the adult relationship's, then the bills, then the shopping, then the meal, then the next day. A mother in pain often learns to postpone herself beyond safety. She becomes capable because incapacity is inconvenient to everyone else.

I became capable.

This would become one of the defining tensions of my life. I could endure a great deal. I could keep going. I could manage, organise, produce, care, write, think, cook, travel, study and make things. That competence saved me many times. It also made the pain less visible to others. A woman who continues is often mistaken for a woman who is fine.

I was not fine. I was simply busy.

Looking back now, Belgium was the point at which the childhood signs became adult consequences. The pain acquired weight, history and economic force. It entered the ordinary tasks of life, and because ordinary tasks must be done, I began the long training that would later become my fifteen-minute life. I did not yet call it that. I simply learned that the body had limits, that those limits could be pushed but not erased, and that every action had a price.

The raised shoe did not help me. The wooden mules did not help me. Being told that childbirth explains backache did not help me. What would have helped was curiosity.

That is what I did not receive.

The young mother in Ghent did not need a theory of posture. She needed someone to take the whole body seriously. She needed someone to understand that a trained dancer who says a movement is impossible may be reporting anatomy, not attitude. She needed someone to know that a congenital anomaly at the lumbosacral junction can shape hips, gait, pain, load and function. She needed someone to look three centimetres to the right.

Instead, I was given three centimetres of shoe.

2

Vegetable Soup and Invisible Splinters

When medical doctors consistently dismissed the problem, I did what many people with chronic pain eventually do. I went elsewhere.

This is often described as if it were irrational. It is not. A person in pain does not turn to alternative practitioners because she has lost all reason. She turns to them because the official routes have failed to produce either relief or curiosity. When one doctor after another looks briefly, speaks confidently and sends you away with nothing useful, the field of possible help expands. You begin to look wherever there is a door, a sign, a recommendation, a story, a rumour, a person who once helped somebody else.

At the time, there was not much around. The world had not yet become the wellness marketplace it is now. There were no online forums, no search engines, no patient groups, no Facebook communities, no YouTube explanations, no medical papers available at the click of a button. There were doctors, physiotherapists, chiropractors, homeopaths, healers, rumours and courage. I had to use what was available.

One homeopathic practitioner prescribed vegetable soup.

He gave me the recipe. I followed it. I ate the soup until the smell of it almost made me vomit. This was before I became the kind of cook who could turn ordinary ingredients into something beautiful, before food became one of the ways I brought form, pleasure and order into life. This soup had none of that. It was treatment disguised as food. It was earnest, watery hope in a bowl.

I ate it because I wanted to believe that something simple could help. A recipe is at least a set of instructions. It says: do this, then this, then this. Chronic pain offers the opposite. It is disorder without explanation. A recipe gives the illusion of sequence, and sequence is comforting when the body has become chaotic.

The soup did not help.

Another practitioner was a seer. He told me there were invisible splinters in my body. He pulled them out with his hands. This cost around a hundred dollars. I do not know what he believed he was doing. Perhaps he believed in his own performance. Perhaps he knew exactly what he was doing. Either way, I was the one in pain and I was the one who paid.

Invisible splinters. There is something almost literary about the phrase. It sounds as though it belongs in a fairy tale, somewhere near the red linen copy of *Grimm's Fairy Tales* I had once balanced on my head. A child is cursed with invisible splinters. A healer draws them out. The pain leaves the body. The child walks freely into the forest.

Life, however, is often less well structured than a fairy tale. The splinters were invisible because they were imaginary. The pain remained because the cause was real.

A chiropractor then produced another explanation. I was clenching my teeth, he said, and that was causing the pain in my back. He made me come back twice a week for a year. Each treatment lasted less than five minutes.

This was an efficient business model. It was not an efficient treatment.

I have thought often about the relationship between confidence and error. The more doubtful a practitioner should have been, the more certain he often appeared. This was true among the obvious quacks, but it was not confined to them. The medical doctors were not much better. Their confidence astonished me. They knew so little about what was happening in my body, yet their manner suggested that nothing important had been missed. Their lack of curiosity was the most damaging part.

Curiosity might have saved me years.

Curiosity would have asked why a young woman with a long history of bodily asymmetry had severe lower back pain. Curiosity would have asked why the pain began so young and persisted. Curiosity would have asked why a trained dancer could perform some difficult movements and found others anatomically impossible. Curiosity would have asked whether a raised shoe might have worsened an underlying structural problem. Curiosity would have asked whether the hip, pelvis and spine were telling one story rather than several small unrelated ones.

Instead, I was given explanations.

This is what happens to many people with chronic pain. The explanation comes before the investigation. The patient describes pain. The practitioner selects a familiar category. The body is then made to fit the category. If the category is muscular, the body is stretched. If the category is postural, the body is corrected. If the category is emotional, the mind is interrogated. If the category is spiritual, the soul is instructed. If the category is dental, the teeth are blamed. If the category is invisible splinters, the hands move theatrically through the air and extract nothing.

The patient becomes the site of other people's theories.

At first, I tried to be open. I was young enough to believe that an answer might arrive from an unexpected direction. I had already been taught by my own body that reality does not always fit official categories. Dance had taught me that the body has secret laws. Motherhood had taught me that endurance is not theoretical. Pain had taught me that ordinary language is inadequate. It was therefore possible, for a while, to believe that someone outside mainstream medicine might see what doctors had missed.

There is nothing shameful in that. Desperation should not be confused with stupidity. I was searching because I had to search. I had small children, work, housekeeping, a body that hurt, and no explanation that made sense. In that situation, any confident person offering a theory acquires a certain power. The offer itself becomes seductive. Here is a cause. Here is a method. Here is something to do.

A body in pain wants something to do.

What I did not yet understand was that every wrong theory carries a cost beyond the money paid. The cost is also conceptual. Each wrong theory teaches you to misunderstand yourself in a new way. The vegetable soup suggests that the body can be corrected by purity or discipline. The invisible splinters suggest that the body is invaded by mysterious forces. The teeth theory suggests that the pain originates somewhere far away from the site of suffering. The repeated dismissal by doctors suggests that the pain may be exaggerated, psychological, ordinary, or simply not interesting.

Over time, these theories accumulate. They do not replace one another neatly. They pile up. A person becomes cluttered with explanations. Perhaps it is posture. Perhaps it is childbirth. Perhaps it is shoes. Perhaps it is teeth. Perhaps it is stress. Perhaps it is old emotion. Perhaps it is poor movement. Perhaps it is muscle memory. Perhaps it is weakness. Perhaps it is too much effort. Perhaps it is too little effort. Perhaps it is my fault.

That last sentence is where the damage settles.

A pain without a name easily becomes a defect of character. If nothing can be found, and the pain continues, the patient begins to carry the suspicion that she is somehow producing it herself. This suspicion is rarely stated plainly. It arrives by implication, in tone, in brevity, in the impatience of a consultation, in the cheerful confidence of someone who has not listened properly. It arrives when a practitioner talks past the pain and towards his own theory. It arrives when the body is treated as unreliable evidence.

I now know that my body was reliable evidence from the beginning. It was the interpretations that were unreliable.

At the time, however, I did not have that knowledge. I had pain. I had young children. I had a household. I had work. I had the ordinary pressure of having to continue. Continuing can look like acceptance from the outside. It is often nothing of the kind. It is simply the absence of another option.

I learned to live with pain and on courage alone.

That phrase sounds dramatic, but the life itself was not dramatic most of the time. It was repetitive. Chronic pain often hides inside repetition. It is there when one lifts a child, washes a cup, reaches for a saucepan, bends to pick up toys, walks to the shop, stands in a queue, sits in a car, folds washing, turns in bed, gets up again. It is there before anyone else notices. It is there after everyone else forgets.

The body becomes a private weather system. Other people ask how you are, and you answer according to the social weather, not the bodily one. Fine. Busy. Tired. Getting there. The real report would be too long. It would require diagrams, memory, history and a willingness from the other person to hear what does not resolve into a simple answer.

Pain also changes time. Before I had language for it, I was already beginning to live in units. How long could I carry this? How long could I stand here? How much could I do before the pain became unmanageable? How much could be postponed? Which task had to be done now?

Which action would cost too much later? I did not yet call this time management. I called it getting through the day.

The later version of my life, the fifteen-minute life, did not appear suddenly in old age. It began here, in the early years of trying to keep a household functioning while doctors and practitioners offered me stories that did not fit. The discipline grew slowly. First as necessity, then as habit, then as method.

There is an advantage in some disadvantages, but it rarely announces itself early. At the time, there was no visible advantage in eating medicinal soup, paying for invisible splinters, or having my teeth blamed for my lower back. There was only waste. Yet even then, something was forming. I was learning how to assess claims. I was learning the difference between confidence and knowledge. I was learning that a system can look authoritative while failing to ask the basic question. I was learning that professional language does not guarantee professional insight.

Those lessons would later shape my work as a legal scholar and publisher. They would shape my suspicion of narrow systems, my attention to what is left outside the frame, and my impatience with institutions that confuse procedure with truth. But at that point, I was not thinking in those terms. I was simply a young woman with a back that hurt, moving from one explanation to the next.

The strange thing is that I remained open. I did not become immediately cynical. I kept searching. This was partly hope, partly stubbornness, partly necessity. The pain was too large to ignore, and the official answers were too small to live with. Somewhere, I thought, there had to be a person who could look properly.

That person did not appear in Belgium.

Instead, life moved again. Belgium was economically depressed in the 1980s, and Japan offered work. Tokyo was in its boom years, alive with possibility, movement, money and intensity. We went there because there was work there. I loved Tokyo and I loved my work there.

The pain came too.

3

Tokyo, Boom Years

Tokyo was alive in a way I had not known a city could be alive.

We arrived during the boom years, when Japan seemed to be racing ahead of the rest of the world. Everything moved quickly. Money moved quickly. People moved quickly. Trains arrived with an almost moral precision. Neon filled the streets. Department stores were worlds of their own. Office towers, station platforms, vending machines, restaurants, bookshops, language schools, tiny bars, temples and convenience stores sat inside one another like layers of a civilisation that knew exactly how to function.

I loved Tokyo. I loved the intensity of it, the order, the speed, the strangeness, the work. After the grey heaviness of Europe, Tokyo felt charged. It required alertness. It required attention. It was not a place in which a person could drift. The city trained you to notice: the train line, the exit number, the bow, the correct phrase, the small silence, the packaging, the gesture, the way people carried themselves in crowded spaces without colliding.

In that sense, Tokyo suited me. I have always been attentive to systems, even before I knew that systems would become part of my legal scholarship. A city is a system, and Tokyo was the most disciplined system I had ever entered. It was dazzling, and it was demanding. It asked the body to stand, walk, commute, sit, bow, wait, climb stairs, carry bags, move through crowds and manage exhaustion politely.

My back came with me.

This is one of the dull facts about pain: it migrates faithfully. One can move country, language, climate, profession, relationship and hope, but the body comes too. It enters the new apartment. It sits on the train. It bends to take off shoes. It stands in the queue. It lies awake in the night. It does not care that the city is exciting, or that work is interesting, or that one has begun again.

In Tokyo, as before, I went to doctors. I tried to explain the pain. I tried to describe its force, its pattern, its refusal to behave like an ordinary backache. There were more X-rays, more scans, more professional faces. The result was familiar: nothing serious could be found. Nothing was wrong with my body. Or, more exactly, nothing that they considered relevant could be seen.

That distinction would matter later.

A body can contain something visible that is not interpreted correctly. The failure is then not simply a failure of technology. It is a failure of attention. The image exists, but the meaning does not arrive. A person can be scanned and remain unseen.

At the time, I did not know this. I only knew that the doctors said there was nothing wrong and that the pain continued. That contradiction began to eat into my confidence. If the body is screaming and the images are declared innocent, where is the scream located? If the doctor cannot see the problem, does the problem belong to the patient's imagination? If the pain is real but the explanation is absent, what sort of reality does pain have?

These questions are dangerous because they move quietly from medicine into identity. The patient begins with "Why does my back hurt?" and ends with "What is wrong with me?"

Japan gave me other kinds of practitioners. Some of them were blind. In Japan, blind practitioners have a long history in massage and acupuncture, and I went to several of them. I do not want to romanticise this. They did not solve the problem. But there was something different in the way some of them used their hands. They read the body through touch, not through a screen. They did not stare past me. They did not begin with the assumption that the machine had already said everything worth saying.

This does not mean they diagnosed Bertolotti Syndrome. They did not. Nobody did. But their hands sometimes recognised that something was wrong. Recognition is not the same as cure, but after years of being told that the pain had no visible cause, even partial recognition mattered.

I was also a foreigner, a gaijin, and this shaped everything. Pain is difficult enough in one's own language. In another language it becomes more exposed. I spoke some Japanese and understood more, but I was still outside the structure. I had to enter medical rooms, treatment rooms and social situations without always knowing the rules. I bowed when others bowed. I followed the gestures. I watched carefully. I tried to be acceptable.

A person in pain often becomes excessively agreeable. Pain makes you dependent. Dependence makes you polite. You want the practitioner to like you, to help you, to continue helping you. You do not want to be difficult, hysterical, foreign, demanding, ungrateful or strange. So you make yourself smaller.

I became very good at making myself smaller.

At the same time, my body began to produce episodes that frightened me. I called them attacks. I did not know what they were. I only knew that something happened in my back with such force that the body seemed to collapse around it. It was as though a string had been pulled or plucked deep inside me. The pain came with a sudden violence, followed by weakness, nausea and fear. Sometimes I vomited. Afterwards I was exhausted.

Now, with the diagnosis behind me, I understand these episodes differently. I think my muscles were working too hard to keep me upright and aligned. They had been compensating for the asymmetry and instability of the structure underneath. Eventually, under pressure, they failed. At the time, however, I did not understand anything. I only experienced the attacks as frightening, humiliating and mysterious.

Every attack sent me back into the medical system. More scans. More X-rays. More reassurance. Nothing wrong. Nothing wrong. Nothing wrong.

There are few phrases more maddening to a person in pain.

The phrase is meant to comfort. It does the opposite. If nothing is wrong and the pain is severe, the patient is left alone with an impossible conclusion. Either the doctor has missed something, or the patient is somehow wrong about her own body. When this happens once, it is frustrating. When it happens repeatedly over years, it becomes a form of psychological erosion.

That erosion became anxiety.

I had not begun with anxiety. I had begun with back pain. But after years of crippling pain, repeated medical dismissal, frightening bodily attacks and the implication that the problem was somehow in me rather than in my spine, anxiety entered the picture. It is important to be precise about this. The anxiety was real. It became part of the story. But it was not the origin of the story.

This distinction matters because medicine often reverses the sequence. A person in pain becomes anxious, and then the anxiety is used to explain the pain. The result is circular and cruel. Pain creates fear; fear is then offered as the cause of pain. The structural problem remains untouched.

My anxiety attacks became serious enough that I needed to see a psychiatrist. He was American and, because he could not prescribe medication in Japan, the treatment did not become a pharmacological solution. After a year and a half, the attacks became less frequent. But by then the problem had changed. What had started as backache had become a mental health issue as well.

This is one of the hidden costs of misdiagnosis. It does not merely leave the original condition untreated. It generates secondary damage. Pain produces fear. Dismissal produces self-doubt. Self-doubt produces vigilance. Vigilance produces exhaustion. Exhaustion produces fragility. The patient then arrives at the next consultation carrying not only pain but also the psychological consequences of having been disbelieved.

The next practitioner sees the anxiety and thinks he has found the cause.

In Tokyo, I lived inside this loop. I worked. I loved the city. I studied the language. I tried to function in a place that demanded discipline and attention. I also moved through treatment rooms, medical appointments and private fear. I was capable and frightened at the same time. That combination would later become familiar. Competence on the outside, collapse on the inside. A bright mind managing a body that would not behave.

This is where the later life as a writer, publisher and legal scholar becomes relevant, although I did not know it then. Pain taught me to watch systems from the position of the person they fail. A system can be elegant from the outside and useless to the person whose problem does not fit its categories. Tokyo's trains functioned with precision. The medical pathway did not. The city could move millions of people with astonishing efficiency, but no one could tell me why one woman's back hurt.

The contrast was not lost on me.

I continued searching because searching was the only responsible thing to do. I was not passive. I was not waiting for someone to rescue me while doing nothing. I went to doctors, practitioners, healers, bodyworkers. I paid, explained, undressed, lay down, stood up, followed instructions, returned for appointments, tried to believe and tried not to collapse under disappointment.

Then a friend introduced me to Wakui.

He was a shiatsu practitioner. I entered his room with my pain, as I had entered so many rooms before. My friend introduced us. I bowed. My pain, if it had manners, bowed too.

Wakui spoke no English, but he tried. I told him I spoke some Japanese and understood some more. He gestured for me to lie face-down on the futon. My friend sat on the tatami and stayed in the room. The room was bare, with towels and a futon. I lay down, as instructed.

Then Wakui put his hands into my hip muscles.

I jumped and screamed.

"Bingo!" he said, laughing.

It was not a diagnosis. It was not medicine in the formal sense. It was not a scan, a report, a classification, an injection or a surgical opinion. But it was the closest thing to recognition I had received in years. His hands had found the place. They had found something. They had found enough for him to laugh with the satisfaction of a person who has touched the target.

For a short time, I believed I might have found help.

4

The Onsen Trip

For five months I went to Wakui at least once a week.

His treatment was not gentle. He used his thumbs and fingers as if he meant to enter the body through the muscle. He worked on my hips, lower belly and lower back with an almost alarming force, throwing his body weight into mine. It hurt, but the pain had a different quality from the pain I had lived with for years. It felt purposeful. It felt as if somebody had finally found the place where the body had been guarding itself.

After those sessions I sometimes felt lighter. I cannot say that I was pain-free, because I was not. But something in me seemed to gather itself better. There was a suggestion of core strength where there had been only collapse. That was enough to keep me going back.

Hope rarely arrives as certainty. More often it arrives as a slight improvement. A day that is less bad. A treatment after which one stands a little differently. A practitioner who touches the painful place without flinching, doubting, moralising or explaining it away. After years of being told that nothing was wrong, even temporary relief can feel like the beginning of rescue.

Wakui's practice room was on the second floor. I was twenty-eight years old, yet I climbed those stairs like a much older woman. The room itself was simple: tatami, a futon, towels, a photograph of his wife and children on the windowsill, and the money from sessions placed openly beside it. Sometimes there was a small pile of notes there. He was handsome, funny, married, and the father of two. I liked him. I also knew, because the photograph made it impossible not to know, that he belonged to a family.

That detail matters.

When a patient likes a practitioner, the relationship becomes more complicated. Liking is not romance. It is not trust without boundary. It is not consent to confusion. It is simply human attachment, formed in the vulnerable space where pain is touched and some relief follows. A person who has been dismissed by doctors can become grateful too quickly to someone who appears to understand.

I was grateful.

After about five months, when I was stronger but still not well, Wakui invited me on a trip. Another patient would come too. We would visit an onsen, he said. The hot mineral water might help my back. I told him I had little money because I was attending Nichibei Kaiwa Gakuin, an expensive Japanese language school. I was studying there for three years. He seemed impressed by this, but waved away the problem. He would pay, he said. He called it a medical order.

I did not understand the situation.

There are moments in life when discomfort speaks before the mind can explain it. I felt uncertain. I thought of the money on his windowsill, the photograph of his wife and children, the fact that I was a foreign woman in pain, the fact that he was a practitioner, the fact that another patient would be travelling with us. I wondered whether he was coming on to me. Then I wondered whether I was being suspicious. Then I wondered whether I was being ungrateful. Pain makes people vulnerable, but so does politeness. So does being in another culture. So does being a woman who has learned to keep situations smooth.

He had already bought the tickets. No way back, he said.

So I went.

The next morning I met him on the platform for the bullet train. The other patient was Tanabe, a man seeking relief from symptoms of cancer treatment. He spoke no English and seemed overwhelmed by my presence. I tried to reduce the awkwardness by reducing myself. This had become a habit. In medical rooms, treatment rooms, foreign rooms, male rooms, uncertain rooms, I often made myself smaller.

On the train, Wakui was excited. He pointed out the window, commenting in broken English on clouds, rice fields and whatever else caught his attention. I watched Japan pass by at high speed, the country sliding from city into countryside, from platforms and buildings into fields and mountains. The movement itself had a kind of beauty. I had always been susceptible to the aesthetic force of Japan: the order, the packaging, the attention to form, the precise placement of objects, the way a meal could become a small composition.

Pain did not cancel that. This is another truth often missed in illness narratives. Even when the body is in trouble, the world can remain beautiful. Sometimes beauty becomes sharper because the body is in trouble. A train window, a rice field, the smell of mountain air, a low table set with small dishes, a bowl, a towel, steam rising from water: these things enter memory because the body, frightened and sore, registers them intensely.

When we left the train, we did not go to an inn as I had expected. We went by taxi to a private house deep in the countryside. We opened the windows. The air was cool and smelled of pine. I remember rice fields, people in straw hats, the sound of streams and waterfalls. Then a large, one-storey wooden house appeared behind a gate. Several generations of what seemed to be one large family came out into the garden to greet us. There were very old people, adults our age and children. Wakui seemed to know them all.

This was not the clinical world. It was more intimate, more communal and more confusing.

We were led to a large tatami room, almost empty except for a bright-pink futon. One by one, people received shiatsu. Some were so old and bent that they could barely lie flat. Others sat around the futon talking, laughing, gossiping, holding children, waiting their turn. Wakui was clearly in his element. He moved from back to back, hip to hip, neck to neck, pressing hard, talking quickly, enjoying the attention. He was practitioner, performer, visitor and centre of the room.

When it was my turn, the chatter stopped.

I was the blonde gaijin on the futon, the foreign woman with the painful back, the person everyone could see but perhaps no one quite knew how to place. Silence gathered around the treatment. I lay there while Wakui worked on me. My pain, which had been private for so long, became public in that room. I do not know what the people around me thought. I only remember the strange exposure of it.

After the treatments, we went into another room for dinner. A long, low table had been set. Small dishes appeared in what felt like an endless stream. The food, the arrangement, the low table, the heat of the sake, the voices around me: it was all intimate and bewildering. I did not understand who these people were, how Wakui knew them, what the exact social arrangement was, or what role I had been given inside it.

Because I did not understand, I drank too much.

So did Tanabe and Wakui. The evening moved into the blurred theatre of drunkenness. This was no longer a medical excursion in any ordinary sense. It was food, sake, family, bodies, massage, heat, laughter, obligation and confusion. Eventually we were given a room next to the dining room, where three futons had been rolled out for us.

The next day we were taken to the onsen.

The water was scorchingly hot and smelled strongly of sulphur. I did what I had learned to do in Japan: I watched, then copied. We placed wet towels on our heads and soaked in the yellow mineral water for hours, breathing heavily in the steam. The heat was almost unbearable. The water, the sulphur, the towels, the huffing and puffing, the strange endurance of it all: it felt as if the body were being cooked back into alignment.

For three days the pattern repeated. Shiatsu. Food. Sake. Onsen. Again. The routine had its own logic, though not one I fully understood. The body was pressed, heated, fed, intoxicated, rested, and returned to heat. It was ancient and absurd, generous and unsafe. I was receiving care and losing clarity at the same time.

Wakui remained vague about his relationship with the household. I never found out who they were to him. Perhaps they were patients. Perhaps friends. Perhaps some arrangement I could not read because I did not know enough of the language, culture or social code. The not-knowing mattered. It kept me dependent on him as interpreter, practitioner and organiser. That dependence sat beneath the trip like a current.

On the fourth night, while Tanabe was sleeping, Wakui rolled into my futon and tried to make love to me.

I whispered that he had a wife and children.

He went back to his own futon and later behaved as if nothing had happened.

My fondness for him disappeared.

The next fact is ordinary and important: I did not confront him. I did not make a scene. I did not demand an explanation. I did not accuse him. I did what I had learned to do too often. I withdrew. I stopped going to his practice. I never heard from him again.

That may sound weak to someone reading from a safe distance. It did not feel simple at the time. I was in Japan. I was a foreigner. He had been helping my pain. He had paid for the trip. He knew the people around us. I was physically vulnerable, emotionally exhausted, and still trained by politeness. I had not yet become the more direct woman I would later become. I was still the pleaser, the yes-woman, the one who smoothed things over and removed herself quietly.

But something had ended.

I threw away his drawing and all the photographs from the trip.

I regret the drawing now, in one sense, because drawings would later become strangely important. A drawing would return years afterwards in another form, through another route, with a force I still cannot easily explain. But at the time, throwing it away was a practical act of rejection. His hands had found something in me. His behaviour had destroyed my trust. I did not want his image, his diagnosis, his trip, or the evidence of my dependence.

So I threw it away.

This was another loss in the long history of losses produced by pain. I lost the possibility of continued treatment with someone whose bodywork had helped me. I lost the drawing. I lost a kind of hope. I lost another practitioner without gaining an explanation. Once again, I was alone with my pain.

After that, my anxiety attacks became worse.

This is where the story can easily be misunderstood. Someone might say the anxiety was psychological, as if that settled the matter. Of course it was psychological. Terror enters the psyche. Dismissal enters the psyche. Pain enters the psyche. Being far from home, dependent on practitioners, told repeatedly that nothing is wrong, and placed in ambiguous situations with men who hold power over one's body: all of that enters the psyche. The mind is not separate from the life it has endured.

But the anxiety was not the origin of the back pain. It was one of the consequences of living with severe pain that nobody properly explained.

Eventually I needed a psychiatrist. He was American and, because he could not prescribe medication in Japan, the treatment was not centred on drugs. After about a year and a half, the attacks became less frequent. By then, however, the problem had expanded. What had started as lower back pain had become a mental health issue as well. This is one of the hidden cruelties of delayed diagnosis: the original pain remains, while secondary suffering accumulates around it.

The medical system then sees the secondary suffering and mistakes it for the cause.

I understand now why the anxiety became so severe. The situation was frightening. My pain was real and disabling. The doctors kept telling me that nothing was wrong. My body was producing attacks so violent that I could vomit or nearly pass out. Each attack led to more scans, more X-rays, more failed interpretation. The gap between the medical version of reality and my bodily reality grew wider and wider until I could no longer stand securely in either world.

That gap is a dangerous place to live.

If you believe the doctors, you must distrust your body. If you believe your body, you must distrust the doctors. Neither position is comfortable. The first makes you feel mad. The second makes you feel abandoned. I moved between the two, trying to be reasonable, trying to be brave, trying to remain functional, trying not to become the difficult foreign woman with the mysterious back and the increasingly frightened mind.

Tokyo had given me beauty, work, language, intensity and adventure. It had also given me a deeper understanding of vulnerability. Pain made me searchable. It sent me into rooms I might otherwise have avoided, towards people I might otherwise not have trusted, into arrangements I did not fully understand. It made me grateful for partial relief and too willing to tolerate ambiguity.

That lesson stayed with me.

Years later, when I looked back over the long chain of practitioners, doctors, therapists and healers, I could see how often pain had forced me into asymmetrical relationships. The practitioner had knowledge, or claimed to have it. I had need. The practitioner stood; I lay down. The practitioner touched; I submitted. The practitioner explained; I tried to understand. The practitioner moved on to the next patient; I went home with the consequences.

The onsen trip did not cure me. It did not diagnose me. It did not give me the answer. It gave me something else: a sharp education in the relationship between pain, dependency and boundary.

It also gave me another image of the body. Not the skeleton poster from childhood. Not the raised shoe in Belgium. Not the invisible splinters. Not the scans that said nothing. This time it was a body in yellow sulphur water, wet towel on the head, steam rising, trying to become well through heat, endurance and imitation. A body being pressed on a pink futon in front of strangers. A body lying awake beside two men in a rural Japanese house, wondering what sort of help had turned into what sort of danger.

That body was mine.

It would still be many years before I could say what was structurally wrong with it. But by then I knew something else with certainty. I knew that pain without diagnosis does not leave a person untouched. It changes judgment. It changes risk. It changes the way one enters rooms, accepts offers, trusts hands, refuses help, and leaves without explanation.

After Wakui, I was again on my own.

5

Wooden Wedges and Wine

When the economic bubble in Japan collapsed in 1992, we returned to Europe and settled in Amsterdam.

The return was practical, but it also carried a kind of defeat. Japan had been intense, difficult, beautiful and frightening. It had given me work, language, friendships, bodywork, anxiety, and a deeper education in vulnerability. It had not given me an answer. The pain came back to Europe with me as faithfully as it had gone to Japan.

I decided to have a full medical check-up once more.

There is a peculiar hope in the word "once". One more attempt. One more set of images. One more professional opinion. One more chance that this time someone will see what others have missed. I had been through enough by then to know better, but pain renews hope in humiliating ways. The body hurts, so the mind searches again.

There were more X-rays and more scans.

I do not remember every appointment. There were too many, and they have merged in memory into a long corridor of waiting rooms, examination tables, hard chairs, forms, referrals, explanations, disappointments and shoes put back on after nothing had been solved. What I remember is the pattern. The body hurt. The images did not produce the right meaning. A practitioner offered a method. I tried the method. The pain remained.

This time I was referred to a manual therapist.

She said, "We don't know why it works, we just know that it works."

That sentence should have worried me more than it did. But by then I had heard so many confident explanations that a little uncertainty almost seemed honest. The manual therapist did not pretend to understand the mechanism. She had a technique. She believed in it. I wanted relief.

She used wooden wedges and hammers.

The treatment had the atmosphere of carpentry. My body was positioned, adjusted, wedged and struck into order. It was not exactly violent, but it was mechanical. The spine became an object to be corrected by leverage and force. I lay there while the treatment was performed, waiting for the moment when something might shift, unlock or release.

It did little or nothing.

This is the point at which chronic pain begins to produce a second life alongside the first. There is the visible life: work, children, shopping, writing, cooking, friends, money, family, the ordinary business of being a person. Then there is the hidden treatment life: appointments, exercises, scans, shoes, devices, explanations, payments, hopes, fatigue, and the private calculation of whether the latest attempt has made things better, worse or merely more expensive.

For a long time, I avoided pain medication.

I did not want to become dependent on tablets. I did not want to dull my mind. I did not want to enter the medical route of prescriptions, side effects, dosage, escalation and surveillance. I had already lost enough confidence in the medical profession to hesitate before handing over more of myself to it. So I did what many people do when they do not trust medication but cannot bear pain unaided.

I drank wine.

In my twenties, I self-medicated with about half a bottle of wine a day. In my thirties, this became a bottle, always in the evenings. In my forties, sometimes more. I can write this plainly now because euphemism does not help. Wine became pain medication. It was legal, available, socially acceptable, and it worked quickly enough to become dangerous.

A glass of wine relaxes the muscles. A second glass softens the edges of the day. A third glass lowers the volume of the body. Pain does not disappear, but the relationship to it changes. The mind moves slightly sideways. The body becomes less insistent. Evening becomes possible.

The problem is that alcohol is a bad doctor. It helps immediately and harms cumulatively. It does not investigate. It does not heal. It does not ask why the pain is there. It simply lends temporary relief at a rate of interest that rises with time.

I knew this.

I also knew that the pain was there every day.

This is the sort of contradiction that outsiders sometimes judge too easily. People like clean distinctions: healthy coping, unhealthy coping; good choices, bad choices; discipline, weakness. Chronic pain does not operate inside such tidy categories. It wears down the distance between what one believes and what one does to get through the evening. A person can know that something is not sustainable and still depend on it, because the alternative is another night inside an untreated body.

I eventually stopped drinking alcohol entirely in my early fifties. But before that, wine had carried some of the weight that doctors had left with me. I do not romanticise it. It was self-medication. It was also an indictment of the failure to diagnose and treat the underlying condition.

After I stopped drinking, pain medication became the only option left.

I took as little as possible, mainly Diclofenac. Even then, the body objected. Eventually it caused a rash on my arms and legs. Another remedy became another problem. That is the arithmetic of chronic illness: the treatment has a cost, the absence of treatment has a cost, and the person in pain must continually decide which cost can be paid today.

By then, the financial cost of the search had become enormous. Not in a dramatic single event, but in accumulation. A consultation here, a treatment there, another practitioner, another device, another pair of shoes, another machine, another book, another promise, another attempt. Money left in small and large amounts over years until the total no longer belonged to the category of health expense. It belonged to the category of property.

The value of a large house. That is how I came to think of it.

Later, I would try to calculate it more carefully and arrive at a rough figure of approximately $1.2 million. The number is approximate and should not be treated as an audited financial statement. It includes doctors, specialists, therapists, alternative practitioners, medication, special shoes, exercise regimes, machines, books, travel, equipment, lost opportunities, reduced earning capacity and the thousands of small adjustments that chronic pain forces into a life.

Still, the phrase that comes back to me is simpler: a large house.

There were books, inversion tables, exercise balls, stretchers, massage machines, EMS machines, belts, special shoes and strange contraptions. Some were sensible. Some were desperate. Some were absurd. Some helped briefly. Most did not. The object itself was never the whole point. The purchase was hope made material. A machine in the corner says: perhaps this will help. A new belt says: perhaps this will hold me together. A special shoe says: perhaps the asymmetry can be corrected. A book says: perhaps somebody has understood this before me.

A house bought with pain is not built all at once. It is built from invoices.

The strangest thing is that while all this was happening, I was still living. I was not lying in a dark room doing nothing. I was raising children, working, moving countries, learning languages, reading, writing, cooking, thinking, and trying to remain myself. The pain did not replace life. It infiltrated it. It entered the kitchen, the study, the bedroom, the street, the desk, the relationship, the school meeting, the manuscript, the dinner, the walk to the shops.

I have always cooked. Cooking is one of the ways I understand the world. It is practical and aesthetic at the same time. It requires timing, sequence, attention, judgement and care. It also requires standing, bending, lifting, reaching and cleaning up afterwards. For most people, those actions are background. For me, they slowly became the physical infrastructure of pain.

Even then, I did not want to give up the kitchen. A meal is evidence that life has not been reduced to symptoms. To cook is to insist on taste, smell, colour, texture and hospitality. It is to make something generous out of limitation. But cooking with back pain is also a negotiation. What can be chopped sitting down? What can be prepared earlier? How long can I stand at the stove? What can be done in one sequence to avoid walking back and forth? Which saucepan is too heavy? Which dish will require too much washing up? When should I stop before the pain takes revenge?

These calculations would become more explicit later, but they began long before I named them. The fifteen-minute life was already forming inside the ordinary life.

Writing was similar. A page does not care whether the writer is sitting properly. It requires attention, not posture. That is one reason writing became possible when other things became harder. It could be done in fragments. It could be done lying down. It could absorb pain without asking the body to perform elegance. The page was less demanding than the street, the sink or the chair.

Painting was different again. It used the hands, eyes and body differently. It required seeing. It required colour and line. It required the willingness to make marks without knowing exactly where they would lead. Later, my drawings and silhouettes would become another way to speak about the body. But even before that, art offered a form of contact with the world that did not begin with medical explanation.

These creative acts did not cure the pain. That is not their value. Their value was that they refused the total authority of pain. They gave me other forms of evidence about myself. I was not only the woman with the back. I was a mother, writer, cook, artist, reader, worker, traveller and thinker. I had a body that hurt, but I also had a mind that kept moving.

This is one reason I dislike the phrase "pain identity". It is often used as if people in chronic pain cling to pain because it gives them a role. In my experience, the problem is often the opposite. The person in pain must work very hard to prevent the pain from swallowing all the other identities. Pain is greedy. It wants the whole room. It wants the schedule, the money, the attention, the relationship, the profession, the imagination and the future. To keep making things under those conditions is not attachment to pain. It is resistance.

Amsterdam gave me no solution. The wooden wedges did not work. The hammers did not work. The scans did not produce the answer. Wine worked too well and not well enough. Diclofenac helped only at a cost. The machines and devices accumulated. The hidden house of pain grew more expensive.

And still, from the outside, a life continued.

This is one of the hardest truths for people without chronic pain to grasp. A person can be functioning and failing at the same time. She can send the email, cook the meal, write the chapter, attend the appointment, raise the children, do the work, meet the friend, and then collapse where no one sees her. The public act is mistaken for the whole condition. It is not. It is often only the visible tip of a much larger strategy.

By the end of the Amsterdam years, I understood that Europe had not given me an answer any more than Japan had. The explanations had changed language and technique, but the structure of failure remained the same. The wrong thing was being treated. Or, more accurately, many possible secondary things were being treated while the primary structure remained unnamed.

A manual therapist could hammer wedges under me. A doctor could prescribe medication. A device could stretch me. A bottle of wine could numb me. A book could persuade me to try another theory. None of it answered the question that had been present since childhood.

What is wrong with my body?

In 2000, I moved again, this time to Australia. It fulfilled a lifelong dream. I was single again. No relationship had survived the pressure of ongoing pain. My children were adults. I entered the country with hope, because hope is persistent even when it has been humiliated.

Australia seemed to me an enlightened country. Perhaps there, finally, someone would know.

6

The Enlightened Country

In 2000, I moved to Australia.

It had been a lifelong dream. Australia existed in my imagination as a place of light, space and possibility. It was far from Europe, far from Japan, far from the accumulated failure of previous medical explanations. I arrived single again. No relationship had survived the pressure of ongoing pain. My children were adults. The shape of my life had changed, and I was ready for a new country to mean a new beginning.

That is one of the temptations of migration. Geography offers the fantasy of renewal. One imagines that a different climate, a different health system, a different culture and a different sky might alter the terms of the body. Australia had good doctors, good hospitals, good public systems, and a reputation for practicality. I thought of it as an enlightened country. Perhaps, at last, someone there would know what had been missed.

The pain did not respect the fantasy.

I entered the mainstream medical maelstrom again. There were more appointments, more attempts to explain, more cautious optimism, more disappointment. The Australian health care system had many strengths, and I do not deny them. Still, it had no explanation for my back pain. It had no solution. I kept having backache attacks, followed by extreme weakness and fatigue. The pattern was now familiar: the body failed, I searched for help, and the answer retreated.

At first, I lived in New South Wales. There, a chiropractor told me that my backache almost certainly came from my cheek joints. The muscles around these joints were extremely tense, he said. The explanation was not new. I had already heard a version of it. My teeth, my jaw, my face, my tension, my clenching: all of them had been given their turn as suspect.

I let him treat me for about a year.

That sentence deserves to be read slowly. I let him treat me for about a year. Chronic pain does that to a person. It stretches the patience beyond reason. A treatment that might have seemed absurd from a distance becomes tolerable because the person offering it appears confident and the alternative is to return to nothing. Week after week, one submits to the method. Week after week, one waits for evidence that the theory is right. Week after week, the money and time leave. At some point, the patient becomes less a believer than an investor. Having spent so much, she wants the explanation to become true.

It did not.

There was no improvement.

In Nimbin, a couple practising Ayurvedic medicine danced around me while I lay face down with a pile of warm chickpea dough on my back.

That sentence needs very little embellishment. It contains its own argument.

The warm dough sat on my back. The practitioners moved around me. I lay there, compliant and sore, inside yet another system of meaning. There is something almost comic about the scene now, though it was not comic then. Pain is good at making the ridiculous seem plausible. It widens the acceptable range of interventions. The more official medicine fails, the more available the unofficial becomes. A woman with a chronic, unnamed pain will eventually tolerate almost anything if it arrives with sufficient seriousness.

I had already eaten the homeopathic vegetable soup. I had paid for invisible splinters to be removed. I had worn the raised shoe. I had submitted to wedges, hammers, machines, belts, exercises, hands, needles, theories and corrections. Warm chickpea dough was another entry in the archive.

I do not tell these stories to mock alternative medicine as a whole. That would be too simple. Some practitioners outside mainstream medicine have touched the body with more attention than doctors who spent less than ten minutes dismissing it. Some helped temporarily. Some recognised distress where the official system saw an inconvenience. The problem lies elsewhere. Pain without diagnosis produces a market. Around that market gather competent people, kind people, deluded people, exploitative people and people who have mistaken their method for truth.

The patient must navigate them while exhausted.

During these years, I also travelled to New York and visited Dr John Sarno's back pain clinic. I had read Sarno's books eagerly. He argued that many chronic back pain conditions were caused by suppressed anger and other repressed emotions. The condition was called Tension Myositis Syndrome, or TMS. To a person who had received no convincing structural diagnosis, the theory had a certain force. Perhaps this was the answer. Perhaps the pain came from the brain. Perhaps the bones and muscles were secondary. Perhaps the body was staging a distraction from emotional truth.

I wanted the theory to work.

I did not approach it lazily. I studied it. I read Sarno and then read other TMS practitioners. I took the idea seriously because I had learned to take every possible answer seriously. I journalled. I wrote down my entire life story in search of possible youth trauma. I talked to my brain for years. I said things to it like: Brain, take away the pain. You have put it there. You can take it away.

This was not casual experimentation. It was disciplined hope.

I also studied Buddhism for several years and became a mindfulness and meditation instructor. I stayed in a Buddhist monastery for six months. Twice a day, I sat cross-legged for two hours. While I sat, I wondered why my right side hurt so much.

This is the part of the story that should put an end to the claim that I had failed to examine the psychological or spiritual dimensions of pain. I examined them intensely. I meditated. I watched sensation arise and pass. I studied the mind. I practised stillness. I learned to sit with discomfort, breath, attention and discipline. I learned the language of awareness. I learned that the mind can enlarge suffering and sometimes soften it. I also learned that a malformed spine does not become normally formed because the mind has become more observant.

Buddhist practice gave me many things. It gave me tools of attention. It gave me a way to observe thoughts without immediately becoming them. It gave me a calmer relationship with some forms of fear. It gave me discipline. It did not remove the structural cause of my pain.

The TMS theory now appears to me far more dangerous for people with Bertolotti Syndrome than it appeared then.

The danger is specific. Bertolotti Syndrome is a congenital structural condition. The pain, where it is symptomatic, arises from abnormal bony anatomy, altered biomechanics, pseudo-joints, bone-on-bone contact, inflammation, nerve irritation, compensatory strain or related structural consequences. A person with this condition does not need to be persuaded that the spine is irrelevant. She needs the spine to be properly examined.

TMS directs attention away from the structure. It encourages the sufferer to stop looking at scans, stop seeking bodily explanations, stop "feeding" the pain with attention, and look instead for repressed anger, psychological conflict, fear of pain or attachment to pain identity. For some people with other kinds of pain, such work may be meaningful. For a person whose lower spine contains an abnormal structure that has been missed for decades, it can be disastrous.

It delays diagnosis.

It also shifts responsibility onto the patient. If the pain continues, the implication is that the sufferer has failed at the psychological work. She has not journalled honestly enough. She has not faced her anger. She remains too attached to the pain. She is too frightened, too invested, too identified, too resistant, too unconvinced. The body disappears again, this time under a language of psychological insight.

That can become another form of gaslighting.

I use the word carefully. Gaslighting occurs when a person's reality is systematically displaced by another version of events imposed with confidence. In the medical context, the effect can be devastating. A patient says: my back hurts, my body is failing, something is wrong. The response is: your body is safe, the pain is generated by the mind, further investigation will reinforce your false belief. The patient is then asked to ignore the very evidence that would eventually lead to diagnosis.

For years, I tried to persuade my brain to stop producing pain. My brain, quite sensibly, refused to comply. It had not put a malformed vertebra there. It could not remove it.

This does not mean the mind is irrelevant to chronic pain. It plainly is relevant. Fear, attention, fatigue, trauma, depression, stress and isolation all shape the experience of pain. Long-term pain changes the nervous system. A life lived under bodily threat changes the mind. There is no clean separation between physical and psychological suffering. The issue is sequence and causation. In my case, the pain began with the body. The psychological consequences accumulated around it after years of disbelief, failed treatments and fear.

The TMS framework reversed that sequence.

I carried that reversal for years.

A diagnosis like TMS can be seductive because it offers control. If the brain creates the pain, perhaps the brain can stop the pain. If suppressed anger generates symptoms, perhaps self-knowledge can cure them. If the body is structurally sound, perhaps one can safely push through. The theory converts the terrifying randomness of pain into a moral and psychological project. It gives the sufferer work to do. Work can feel better than helplessness.

I have always been good at work.

So I worked at it. I journalled, meditated, read, attended, reflected, instructed, practised. I sat in the monastery with my legs crossed, trying to make sense of the pain on my right side. I investigated my past. I searched for emotional explanations. I tried to stop being afraid. I tried to believe that nothing was structurally wrong.

The body kept insisting.

There is a deep irony here. The same discipline that made me a writer, cook, publisher, painter and legal scholar also made me vulnerable to difficult theories. I do not abandon a problem easily. Give me a method and I will test it properly. Give me a theory and I will read the books. Give me an exercise and I will do it. Give me a discipline and I will apply myself. That persistence has served me well in many parts of life. It has also kept me too long inside systems that were not helping me.

Australia taught me that the enlightened country was still a country of human beings, and human beings carry their blind spots into every profession. A chiropractor can blame the cheek joints. An Ayurvedic couple can dance around chickpea dough. A famous doctor can send pain into the unconscious. A meditation practice can teach attention without solving anatomy. A good health system can still miss a condition its practitioners have not been trained to look for.

The problem was not that nobody cared. Some did care. The problem was that caring without the right conceptual frame has limited use. A practitioner can be kind and wrong. A doctor can be competent and incurious. A theory can be elegant and misapplied. A system can be well-funded and still fail the person whose condition sits outside its usual categories.

I was beginning to understand this long before I had the legal language for it.

Later, as a legal scholar, I would become interested in systems, categories, blind spots and the consequences of institutional attention. Who gets seen? Who gets classified? Who gets believed? Who is forced to translate lived reality into a language the system recognises? Who pays when the category is wrong? Those questions did not begin in a library. They began in my body.

The body is a strict teacher.

By then, I had become skilled at searching. I searched medical literature, popular health books, alternative systems, spiritual traditions, therapeutic explanations and my own past. I had searched in Europe, Japan, the United States and Australia. The search had made me resourceful. It had also made me tired.

I moved to Alice Springs in 2004.

Central Australia had its own intensity: red earth, heat, distance, light, dryness, sky. It was beautiful and severe. I would live there for many years. I would write, work, study law, build a community, found a publishing house, complete a PhD, paint, cook, swim, and organise a life of increasing physical constraint. I would also enter the next stage of the medical ordeal.

By then, the pain had travelled with me through five countries. It had survived doctors, shoes, wedges, hammers, wine, acupuncture, shiatsu, hot springs, chiropractic theories, Ayurvedic dough, TMS, Buddhism, meditation and my most disciplined attempts at self-examination.

It was still unnamed.

7

Central Australia

I moved to Alice Springs in 2004.

Central Australia is not a gentle landscape. It is beautiful, but it does not soothe in the ordinary sense. It exposes. The light is hard, the distances are immense, the air is dry, and the earth is red in a way that seems almost geological rather than decorative. After Europe and Japan, Alice Springs felt spare, direct and severe. There was no mistaking where one was. The place had a physical force.

I liked that.

A body in pain often becomes tired of softness. Soothing language, comforting theories, sympathetic smiles and vague encouragements can become intolerable when they do not lead anywhere. The desert had no interest in pretending. It was not kind, but it was clear. It did not tell me my pain was in my head. It did not tell me to relax. It did not hand me vegetable soup, invisible splinters, wooden wedges or warm chickpea dough. It simply stood there, ancient and indifferent, and required me to live.

I had my back examined again.

By then, I had entered a familiar pattern. I no longer arrived at appointments with the clean optimism of a person seeking help for the first time. I arrived carrying Europe, Japan, New South Wales, Nimbin, New

York, Buddhism, TMS, scans, shoes, practitioners, books, devices, exercises, wine and exhaustion. I also arrived carrying an increasingly accurate private conviction: the problem was real, structural and repeatedly missed.

Private conviction is useful. It is also lonely.

In Alice Springs I had several attacks that led to hospitalisation. The word "attack" was still the best word I had for them. Something would happen in my back with such force that the body seemed to lose its scaffolding. The pain was severe, but the aftermath was often worse: weakness, fatigue and the feeling that the whole muscular system had gone into shock. These episodes were frightening because they did not feel like ordinary flare-ups. They felt like collapse.

In the emergency room, I encountered a doctor who clearly thought I was faking the whole thing.

I do not know what he saw when he looked at me. Perhaps he saw a woman in distress whose scans had not provided an easy emergency explanation. Perhaps he saw another back-pain patient taking up time in a pressured system. Perhaps he saw anxiety and decided the body could therefore be ignored. Perhaps he had been trained, informally if not formally, to distrust pain that did not present in the clean shape expected by emergency medicine.

I know what I felt. I felt the old humiliation return.

To be in severe pain and be suspected of invention is a particular kind of degradation. It places the patient in an impossible position. If she remains calm, the pain cannot be that bad. If she cries, she is emotional. If she insists, she is difficult. If she withdraws, she is evasive. If she knows too much, she is self-diagnosing. If she knows too little, she is unreliable. The medical gaze can turn every response into evidence against the patient.

Later, a visiting spine surgeon labelled the problem myofascial pain syndrome.

I accepted the words because I had no better ones. The phrase sounded technical. It had the comfort of Latin. It moved the problem into muscles and fascia, which was partly plausible. My muscles certainly hurt. My body had spent decades compensating. The hips, back, pelvis and legs were all caught in patterns of strain. But a muscular label did not explain why the muscles were in such trouble. It did not explain the childhood asymmetry, the one-sided dance limitations, the raised hip, the wrong shoe, the attacks, the fatigue, the failure of every theory that had gone before.

It named the smoke and missed the fire.

This is one of the recurring dangers in chronic pain medicine. A secondary effect becomes the diagnosis. The muscles hurt, so the problem is muscular. The patient is anxious, so the problem is anxiety. The patient is tired, so the problem is fatigue. The patient has learned to guard herself, so the problem is guarding. All of these things may be true. None of them necessarily explains the cause.

By then, the ordeal had affected my mind. I developed PTSD, saw both a psychologist and a psychiatrist, and started taking anti-anxiety medication again. This is another fact that must be held in the right order. The mental health consequences were real. They deserve to be taken seriously. But they were consequences of years of severe pain, disbelief, frightening bodily events and failed explanations. They were not the origin of the condition.

The failure to keep that order clear is one of the ways patients are harmed.

I had several X-rays and MRI scans. I did yoga. I bought another generation of equipment from the ever-growing wellness industry. I began juicing. I took supplements. I read everything I could find about lower back pain. The search had become almost professional in its intensity. I was no longer simply a patient following advice. I had become a researcher of my own body.

This would later connect naturally with my life as a legal scholar. Research begins with dissatisfaction. A received answer does not fit the evidence. A category fails. A system produces an unjust or inadequate result. One goes back to the materials, the facts, the assumptions, the language, the gaps. In law, this can become scholarship. In medicine, for the patient, it becomes survival.

Alice Springs was the place where these strands of my life began to gather more closely. I lived with pain, but I also lived as a writer, a thinker, a cook, an artist and a person who needed work to have meaning. The pain did not remove my appetite for life. It made the pursuit of life more complicated.

I still cooked. The kitchen remained one of the places where I could make something coherent. Cooking is a discipline of sequence. It asks for preparation, attention, timing and judgement. It also asks the body to stand, reach, chop, lift, stir, bend and clean. That meant cooking became both pleasure and calculation. I learned to plan the order of tasks more carefully. I learned to prepare what could be prepared sitting down. I learned that even beautiful food has a physical cost. Yet I kept cooking because food is more than nourishment. A good meal says that life has texture. It says that the senses still matter. It says that pain has not taken hospitality.

I painted too. Painting gave me another kind of language. It did not ask me to explain myself to a doctor. It did not demand proof. It allowed form, colour, line and mood to carry what ordinary words could not. Later, my silhouettes would make the asymmetry of the body visible in a way medical encounters had failed to do. Art has this advantage: it can show what a report does not say.

Writing remained the most durable practice. The page was patient. It allowed interruption. It allowed return. It did not require me to stand in a queue, sit in a hard chair, or walk further than the body permitted. Writing could be done in fragments, and fragments were increasingly the unit in which life had to be lived. A paragraph could be written lying down. A poem could form around pain without becoming a medical document. A sentence could remain alive even when the body was not cooperating.

That mattered.

People often assume that chronic pain narrows a person into the role of patient. In practical terms, it tries to. It takes time, money, movement, sleep, attention and confidence. It fills diaries with appointments and homes with devices. It distorts work and relationships. But a person is not obliged to surrender the whole self to the category of illness. I did not want to become only the woman with the back. I was, and remained, a writer, a painter, a cook, a reader, a mother, a friend, a publisher in formation, and eventually a legal scholar.

This did not mean I was coping well. It meant I was refusing erasure.

The distinction matters. Productivity is often misunderstood as evidence of wellness. If I could write, I must be all right. If I could cook, I must be exaggerating. If I could paint, study or discuss ideas, perhaps the pain was manageable. That is not how chronic pain works. Many people function by borrowing from the next day, or the next week, or the next decade. The task is done. The cost is paid later, privately.

I became skilled at paying privately.

Alice Springs also brought community. A remote town has its own intensity. People know one another. Lives overlap. News travels. Friendships can become practical in a way that city friendships sometimes are not. For a person living with chronic pain, practical friendship matters more than sympathy. Sympathy says, "That must be awful." Practical friendship says, "Lie down; I'll make the tea," or "I'll carry that," or "Let's meet somewhere with a couch," or "I understand if you need to leave."

There were people who understood, and people who did not. That, too, is part of chronic illness. The social world divides itself according to capacity for adjustment. Some people need the sick person to behave in a way that suits their idea of sickness. If she is too articulate, too funny, too productive or too well dressed, they become sceptical. Others understand that suffering does not always look like collapse. Those are the people one keeps.

By the time I had seen ten, twenty or thirty therapists, doctors, masseurs and chiropractors in Alice Springs, my GP finally placed me on the waiting list for the pain clinic at Alice Springs Hospital.

It took a year before my name reached the top.

A year is a long time in pain. It is long enough to try several more theories. Long enough to buy more equipment. Long enough to read more books. Long enough to worsen, recover slightly, worsen again and invent new forms of adaptation. Long enough to become older. Long enough to ask whether the answer, if it ever comes, will arrive too late.

Waiting lists have a moral dimension. They are not merely administrative. They allocate time, and time is not neutral when a person is deteriorating. A year for a healthy person is twelve months. A year for a person in severe pain can be a structural event. Muscles weaken. Fear deepens. Work changes. Social life shrinks. Money drains. Hope becomes harder to keep clean.

During that year, I kept searching.

I turned again to the edges of medicine and meaning. I took mushrooms and ayahuasca with one question in mind: what is wrong with my back? That may sound reckless to some readers and understandable to others. I had been asking doctors that question for decades. I had asked physiotherapists, chiropractors, bodyworkers, healers, psychiatrists, books, Buddhist practice and my own mind. The question remained open. At some point, a person begins to ask reality itself.

I also took somatic healing classes, and those helped me. I say this carefully because I do not want to replace one false universal answer with another. Somatic healing did not diagnose Bertolotti Syndrome. It did not correct the anatomy. It did help me deal with pain. It helped me listen to the body without making the body guilty. It gave me ways to reduce fear, soften vigilance and inhabit sensation without immediately turning it into catastrophe. That is valuable.

The test for any method, in my view, is whether it helps without lying. A method can be useful if it relieves suffering, improves function, supports attention or reduces fear. It becomes dangerous when it claims to explain everything, dismisses structural causes, or tells the patient that continuing pain is proof of psychological failure.

By that stage of life, I had become wary of total explanations. That wariness was earned.

I had also begun to understand how pain had trained my mind. It had trained me to look for hidden structures. It had trained me to distrust confident surface accounts. It had trained me to ask who benefits when a category is accepted too quickly. It had trained me to notice what a system refuses to see. These habits would become useful in legal scholarship. They also kept me alive as a patient.

The law, like medicine, depends on classification. A person becomes a tenant, patient, offender, victim, complainant, applicant, respondent, scholar, disabled person, difficult person, non-specific back-pain sufferer. Categories are useful because systems cannot operate without them. Categories are dangerous because they can become substitutes for attention. Once the category is applied, the person may disappear.

I had disappeared many times under categories. Postural problem. Leg-length discrepancy. Myofascial pain. Anxiety. TMS. Wear and tear. Chronic back pain. Difficult patient. Woman in pain. Too complicated.

None of those categories was the name of the thing.

Alice Springs gave me years of work, friendship, study, cooking, writing, painting and community. It also gave me hospitalisation, humiliation, psychiatric injury, waiting lists, and another layer of medical exhaustion. The two truths belong together. A place can nourish a life and fail a body. A person can build community while becoming more physically restricted. A woman can make books, meals, paintings and legal arguments while still needing help to stand, sit, walk and recover.

This is why the story must be told whole. Pain is central, but it is not sovereign. It shaped the life. It did not own all of it.

The year on the waiting list eventually ended. My name reached the top. I went to the pain clinic, carrying decades of wrong explanations, a body that was almost out of patience, and a drawing I had nearly stopped believing.

The doctor there was a warm, kind woman from India.

She would ask me one question that changed the story:

"Do you know what you have?"

8

Sit Down, Dear

By the time my name reached the top of the pain clinic waiting list, I was well into my sixties.

This fact still feels strange to write. There is a particular absurdity in arriving at the correct diagnosis near the end of the story, after the body has already spent decades adapting, compensating, deteriorating and defending itself. A diagnosis in youth can redirect a life. A diagnosis in old age explains a life that has already been spent.

During the year of waiting, I had continued to search. I had read, practised, exercised, rested, tried somatic healing and returned, once again, to the central question that had followed me through five countries: what is wrong with my back?

At some point, I turned to mushrooms and ayahuasca. I did so with one specific question in mind. I was not looking for entertainment, revelation, ecstasy or escape. I was not looking for a spiritual decoration to place over an unsolved medical problem. I had lived with pain for nearly five decades. I had asked doctors, physiotherapists, chiropractors, bodyworkers, healers, psychiatrists, meditation teachers, books, machines and my own mind. I had asked nicely and desperately. I had asked in Dutch, English and Japanese. I had asked through obedience, research, discipline and endurance.

The question remained.

What is wrong with my back?

One night on ayahuasca, I entered intense, hallucination-like states. During the trip, a blind Japanese man walked up to me and handed me a drawing.

That image struck me with particular force because of Japan. The blind practitioners I had seen there had held a different place in my memory from most other practitioners. They had not diagnosed me, but their hands had sometimes recognised something. They had read the body through touch rather than through the dismissive logic of an image reported as normal. In the ayahuasca state, this blind Japanese man returned as a figure of recognition. He did not speak. He handed me an image.

The next day, over coffee, I sketched the drawing for my friend Marilyn. This matters because the episode sounds almost unbelievable, and I am wary of unbelievable stories when they are told without witnesses. Marilyn saw me draw it. I announced, with the seriousness of someone who has just been handed a message by a plant and a blind Japanese doctor from the unconscious, "The Plant has spoken. It said this."

The drawing showed my L5 vertebra with butterfly-like wings on each side. One of the wings was connected to the sacrum.

At that stage, I did not know what to do with the image. I did some research and found a possible explanation. Then I went to my GP and said, "I've done some research. I think I have this." I placed the drawing on her desk.

She looked at it and said, "No, what you have is wear and tear of your spine."

Wear and tear. The phrase is one of those apparently harmless medical expressions that can close a door. It has the weary authority of age. It suggests that the body is simply old, used, frayed, ordinary in its decline. It does not invite curiosity. It tells the patient to accept deterioration as natural, expected and mostly uninteresting.

By then I was tired enough to believe her, or at least to stop arguing. I had long since learned that the patient's certainty is rarely welcomed unless it arrives from the right direction. If a doctor says "wear and tear", the phrase becomes respectable. If a patient places a drawing on the desk and says, "I think this is my spine", she risks becoming the difficult patient, the self-diagnoser, the woman who has read too much and misunderstood it.

So I dismissed what the Plant had told me.

Then came the appointment at the pain clinic.

The doctor was a warm, kind woman from India. I remember her warmth because warmth had not been the dominant mood of my medical journey. Kindness in a clinical room can seem minor to those who have not spent decades being doubted. It is not minor. It changes the air. It allows the patient to speak without immediately armouring herself against dismissal.

She asked me, "Do you know what you have?"

I answered with the phrase I had been given. "Wear and tear on my spine."

She said, "Sit down, dear."

Then she took an A4 sheet of paper and began to draw.

I watched her hand move across the page. I had seen so many diagrams over the years, so many vague gestures towards discs, muscles, posture, joints, fascia, nerves and tension. But this drawing was different. It was not a generic spine. It was not the usual explanatory sketch practitioners make when they are trying to simplify the body for a patient. It was exact in the only way that mattered. It matched the image I had seen in the trip. It matched the drawing I had made for Marilyn. It showed the L5 vertebra with its abnormal wings, one of them connected to the sacrum.

Next to the drawing she wrote: Bertolotti Syndrome.

At first, I could not speak.

There are moments when the mind stops because the body has understood before language catches up. The room, the doctor, the page, the chair, the decades, the previous explanations, the child stumbling in the Netherlands, the dancer with one impossible side, the young mother in Ghent, the raised shoe, the Japanese blind practitioners, Wakui's hands, the onsen, the vegetable soup, the invisible splinters, the wooden wedges, the wine, the chiropractor blaming my cheek joints, the Ayurvedic chickpea dough, Sarno, the monastery, the emergency room doctor who thought I was faking, the visiting spine surgeon, the PTSD, the scans, the waiting list, the ayahuasca drawing: all of it suddenly rearranged itself around a name.

Bertolotti Syndrome.

I started nodding. "Yes," I said. "Yes, that is what it is."

The rest of the visit is a blur. I think I cried a little. Afterwards, I had to sit down for a while because my legs were too weak to walk.

That weakness was not only physical. Something had given way. For almost fifty years I had been carrying an unsolved problem inside a body that other people kept misreading. The diagnosis did not remove the pain, but it removed the accusation that had hovered around it. The pain had not been imaginary. It had not been a failure of character. It had not been unexpressed anger, weak muscles, poor posture, anxiety, old trauma, spiritual ignorance, teeth clenching, a short leg, insufficient discipline, or the ordinary decay of age.

It was anatomy.

Relief is too simple a word for what followed. Relief was there, but so was grief. A correct diagnosis late in life does not return the decades. It does not refund the money. It does not undo the wrong shoe, the unnecessary treatments, the self-doubt, the anxiety, the lost work, the relationships strained by pain, the years spent trying to persuade my brain to stop producing a pain it had never invented. It does not give back the body before compensation became damage.

What it gives is meaning.

Meaning matters. It does not cure, but it changes the relationship to the past. It gathers scattered episodes into a single account. It says that the child's stumbling was data. The one-sided split was data. The groin pain was data. The raised hip was data. The back attacks were data. The fatigue after collapse was data. The failure of psychological explanations was data. The fact that rest helped was data. The fact that pushing through made everything worse was data. The body had been speaking the whole time.

Nobody had known the language.

The doctor prescribed three medications to relax my muscles: Tramadol 50 mg, Amitriptyline Viatris 30 mg and Baclofen 25 mg. I was already taking Mirtazapine 30 mg for anxiety. Together, the drugs were far too much for me. I later described the cocktail as enough to bring down a horse.

I took them for three weeks and then stopped them all.

I now call it chemical rape.

I use that phrase because the experience felt like a violation of the mind and body together. The medication did not merely soften pain. It entered the whole system and altered me. It interfered with the person I knew myself to be. I have always relied on my mind. If the body has been unreliable, the mind has been my place of movement. It has carried writing, painting, scholarship, publishing, cooking, planning, memory, humour and work. To have that mind chemically flattened was frightening. It was another reminder that treatment itself can become harmful when it does not properly take account of the whole person.

This does not mean medication is wrong for everyone. It means that medication, like every other intervention, has to be understood in context. A prescription is not merely a list of substances. It is an event in a person's life. It lands inside a body with history, inside a mind with work to do, inside a household, a business, a set of responsibilities, a long record of medical failure and a particular tolerance for risk. For me, that combination was intolerable.

After the diagnosis, I read and read.

Research had long been a survival strategy. Now it became more focused. The condition had a name. I could search properly. I could read about lumbosacral transitional vertebrae, pseudo-articulations, abnormal transverse processes, diagnostic injections, surgical options, classification systems and the continuing uncertainty around treatment. I could finally enter the literature through the right door.

I learned that I had type 1A.

I also learned that the prognosis was not encouraging. My doctor said I was too old for an operation. That sentence landed with its own finality. Too old. Too late. Too much time gone. The possibility that a younger version of me might have been helped was difficult to bear. I do not know with certainty what would have happened if the diagnosis had arrived earlier. I will not pretend to know. But I do know that earlier recognition would have spared me decades of wrong explanations and dangerous detours. It would have given me informed choices.

That is no small thing.

A person does not need a guaranteed cure to benefit from a correct diagnosis. A correct diagnosis allows proper caution. It allows targeted treatment. It allows better questions. It allows the person to stop injuring herself in the name of false reassurance. It allows rest to be understood as protection rather than weakness. It allows pain to be interpreted as information rather than hysteria. It allows the patient to stop apologising for the body's limits.

This was the greatest practical change. I no longer had to obey theories that contradicted my body. I no longer had to push through pain because someone had told me that the spine was safe. I no longer had to treat rest as failure. I no longer had to wonder whether I had failed to journal honestly enough, meditate deeply enough, relax sufficiently, or face the correct buried emotion.

Bertolotti Syndrome gave me permission to believe my body.

The diagnosis also changed the way I understood my own competence. For years, I had thought of myself as someone who had somehow managed, despite a mysterious back. After diagnosis, I understood the scale of that management differently. I had lived, worked, raised children, migrated, written, cooked, studied, practised meditation, painted, founded a publishing house and completed legal scholarship while carrying a congenital spinal condition that had never been properly treated. What had appeared to others as productivity was often an elaborate act of adaptation.

This recognition was not pride. It was clarification.

It also sharpened my anger. Anger can be useful when it is precise. I was not angry because one doctor had missed one thing on one day. I was angry because an entire pattern of professional attention had failed. The spine had been imaged many times. The body had been examined many times. The patient had spoken many times. The symptoms had begun young, persisted for decades, involved asymmetry, pain with activity, relief with rest, and repeated functional collapse. Yet the relevant structure remained unrecognised until late life.

How many times can a system look at a person without seeing her?

That question belongs to medicine, but it also belongs to law, education, housing, disability policy and every institution that converts lived reality into categories. It is one reason the diagnosis connected so deeply with my legal scholarship. Sustainable Justice, as I came to understand it, requires attention to the structures that shape people's lives. It asks what systems see, what they ignore, whose knowledge counts, and what harm follows when a person is forced into the wrong category. My body had been living that question long before I wrote it academically.

Doctors had looked at my spine, but not three centimetres to the right. That became a metaphor for almost everything.

The problem was not invisibility alone. Bertolotti Syndrome is not invisible in the literal sense. The anatomy can be seen if the viewer knows to look, knows what the structure means, and understands that a transitional vertebra may be clinically significant rather than incidental. The condition was visible but uninterpreted. That is a more unsettling failure. It means the evidence may have been present while the conceptual frame was absent.

Once I had the name, I began to place the past inside the new frame. The child with *Grimm's Fairy Tales* on her head. The dancer with the impossible right side. The young mother given a raised shoe. The woman in Japan whose back attacks were treated as mystery. The patient told that anxiety explained what pain had produced. The believer in TMS talking sternly to her brain. The woman in Alice Springs waiting a year for a pain clinic appointment. They were all the same person, moving through the same undiagnosed condition.

That is what a diagnosis can do. It makes the self continuous.

Before diagnosis, the story had been fragmented into episodes: childhood clumsiness, childbirth backache, leg-length discrepancy, teeth clenching, muscular pain, anxiety, myofascial syndrome, wear and tear. After diagnosis, the fragments formed a line. It did not make the line painless. It made it legible.

Legibility is not everything, but after nearly fifty years, it is a great deal.

I left the pain clinic that day with a name, a drawing, prescriptions I would soon abandon, and a new relationship to my own past. I also left with the knowledge that the name had arrived late. That doubleness has never gone away. Gratitude and anger. Relief and grief. Validation and loss. Recognition and the possibility that recognition had come after the best window for intervention had closed.

A diagnosis can be both a door and a wall.

For me, it was both.

9

Sovereign Health

After the diagnosis, people might assume that the next thing was treatment.

That would have been a natural order: name, plan, intervention, improvement. Medicine likes that sequence. Patients like it even more. It offers the comfort of direction. For almost fifty years I had wanted an explanation; once the explanation arrived, it seemed reasonable to expect the road to open. A named condition should lead somewhere.

Instead, the road narrowed.

My doctor said I was too old for the operation that might help. The sentence was short, and it did what short sentences can do: it closed a door without much ceremony. I understood the logic. Surgery on an older spine carries risk. By then my body had been compensating for decades. Muscles, joints, nerves, posture, gait, balance and endurance had all reorganised themselves around the abnormal structure. I was no longer the young mother in Ghent with two babies and a back that had just begun to speak loudly. I was a woman in her sixties whose body had spent nearly half a century arranging itself around pain.

Even so, the words were difficult to absorb.

Too old. Too late. Too damaged. Too complicated. The exact phrase mattered less than the implication. There might once have been a moment when intervention could have altered the course of things. That moment had passed, or may have passed. I do not know that with certainty. I do know that no one gave me the opportunity to consider it properly when I was younger.

That is one reason delayed diagnosis is not a small matter. It is not merely a delay in naming. It is a delay in choice. If a condition is identified early, a person can decide with knowledge: conservative management, targeted injections, surgery, restraint, monitoring, specialist review, second opinion. Some choices may still be difficult. Some may still fail. But they are choices made in the presence of the right question. Without diagnosis, life becomes a long sequence of decisions made inside the wrong frame.

I had made nearly all my decisions inside the wrong frame.

I had stretched, strengthened, meditated, journalled, analysed, prayed, swum, walked, sat, stood, lifted, rested, blamed myself, forgiven myself, changed shoes, changed countries, changed practitioners, changed diets, changed thoughts, changed beliefs and changed language. I had tried to become more relaxed, more disciplined, more mindful, more physically active, more psychologically honest, less frightened, less identified with pain, less resistant, more open, more accepting.

The diagnosis made much of that labour appear both admirable and absurd. Admirable because I had tried with extraordinary seriousness. Absurd because so much of it was aimed at a body whose structural problem had been missed.

My spine would not be remade.

That became the practical fact. I still had pain, fatigue and weakness. I still had a lopsided body. I still had the aftermath of the medication trial. I still needed a walking stick. I still had to lie flat because lying flat was the only position in which the pain became manageable. I still had ordinary tasks to perform: eating, washing, dressing, cooking, cleaning, answering emails, managing money, running a publishing house, working on books, arranging appointments, maintaining friendships, thinking.

The diagnosis had ended the madness. It had not ended the day.

The first medical response after the diagnosis had been medication. Tramadol, Amitriptyline, Baclofen, and the Mirtazapine I was already taking. The combination changed my body and mind in a way I could not tolerate. My muscles softened too much. My sense of self altered. My mind lost its sharpness. I became someone I did not recognise.

This frightened me because my mind has always been the part of me that could still move.

When the body becomes unreliable, the mind becomes more than intellect. It becomes mobility. It travels where the spine cannot. It makes worlds. It writes books, reads law, follows arguments, solves publishing problems, remembers poems, edits sentences, imagines paintings, plans meals, studies systems, and builds meaning. A mind that can move freely is not a luxury when the body is restricted. It is the remaining country.

The medication threatened that country.

I do not say this as a general argument against medication. Pain medication can be necessary, humane and life-saving. Muscle relaxants may help some people. Antidepressants and anti-anxiety medications can be appropriate. I am not writing a doctrine for others. I am recording what happened in my body. The drugs that were intended to make me more functional made me less myself.

After three weeks, I stopped.

The decision was not romantic. It was practical. I had managed the condition without any real help for forty-eight years. I had not managed it well, because no one can manage an undiagnosed structural condition well. But I had survived it. I had built a life around it. I had developed systems, routines and disciplines. I had used study, reading, meditation, mindfulness and art to keep the mind alive. I had written, painted, cooked, taught myself, published, studied law and completed a PhD. I had made a glowing mind in a wonky body.

Now a doctor whom I might see once every few months for ten minutes wanted to get me "more active".

The phrase had the force of insult, although I do not think it was intended that way. More active. As if activity had been absent from my life. As if I had been waiting passively in a room for medicine to arrive. As if I had not tried everything under the sun. As if the problem were motivational. As if the woman lying flat to work, swimming, using a Pilates reformer, rebounding, cooking, writing, editing books, running a press and thinking all day needed chiefly to be encouraged.

This is another way capable disabled people are misunderstood. Activity is measured by visible movement. If you cannot walk far, stand long or sit comfortably, you may be read as inactive. But there are forms of activity that do not look like exercise. Intellectual work is activity. Creative work is activity. Running a small press is activity. Managing pain is activity. Planning a day around bodily limits is activity. Cooking a meal in stages is activity. Swimming before the body collapses is activity. Resting before damage occurs is also a disciplined form of action.

I no longer accept the idea that activity must look upright.

After the medication episode, I decided to practise what I call Sovereign Health.

The phrase is deliberate. It does not mean rejecting doctors altogether. It does not mean pretending I know everything. It does not mean refusing all treatment, imaging, advice or professional help. It means keeping the final authority over my body as much as possible. It means weighing advice against lived evidence. It means remembering that no practitioner has to live in the consequences of a prescription the way I do. It means refusing to hand my mind and body over to the next confident person with a theory.

I had handed myself over too many times.

Sovereign Health means taking as little medication as possible and keeping my medicine regime in my own hands. It means using professional help selectively rather than obediently. It means listening to my body without turning the body into a god. It means treating rest as information. It means refusing to be pushed into psychological explanations where structural assessment has been inadequate. It means accepting that some methods help without allowing any method to become a religion.

My present regime is modest and repetitive. I have a Pilates reformer in my living room. I have an expensive rebounder with bungee cords. I swim. I go to yoga off and on when I can. These things do not take the pain away. They keep me mobile enough. They keep my core strong enough. They give the day structure. They give the body instructions that are demanding without being destructive.

That distinction matters. Exercise for a body with Bertolotti Syndrome is not a moral virtue. It is a negotiation. Too little movement and the body stiffens, weakens and retreats. Too much movement and it punishes me. The point is not to become fit in the ordinary aspirational sense. The point is to remain possible.

The rebounder helps. The reformer helps. Swimming helps most of all. In water, the body receives a temporary kindness that gravity does not offer. The pool carries some of the load. It allows movement without the same punishment. For a while, I can be almost normal there, or at least less abnormal. My limbs move, my spine is spared some pressure, my breath finds a rhythm, and the body remembers that movement need not always be a threat.

Then I get out of the water and gravity returns.

This is why I do not speak of cures. I speak of management. Management sounds dull, but it is where life happens. A managed condition is still present. It is simply given fewer opportunities to destroy the day.

Management is the art of reducing consequences. It is also the art of preserving what matters.

What matters to me is not simply pain reduction. Pain reduction matters, of course. I would take less pain if it were honestly available. But I also need clarity, creativity, independence, friendship, dignity, language, beauty and work. A treatment that reduces pain but destroys the mind is not acceptable. A therapy that offers hope but requires me to distrust the body is not acceptable. A system that asks me to become passive in exchange for care is not acceptable.

This is where the doctor-patient relationship becomes more complicated than medicine often admits. A patient is not a site for intervention. A patient is a person with a life already in progress. My life includes books, poems, paintings, cooking, publishing and legal scholarship. It includes the discipline of editing other people's sentences, the pleasure of making a meal, the satisfaction of solving a layout problem, the slow architecture of an argument, the intense concentration of writing, the quiet of drawing, the social life of books, the practical joy of sending a manuscript into the world.

None of these can be separated from health.

Health is usually described as if the body were the main object. For me, health has become the capacity to remain myself under constraint. It is the ability to think clearly enough to write. To stand long enough to cook something good. To move enough to swim. To lie down without surrendering. To keep the press running. To answer a friend. To read a difficult text. To have humour left at the end of a day. To make art before pain takes the hand or the back or the concentration.

This is why I am cautious about being made "more active". The phrase is too crude for the life I actually live. I do not need general activity. I need precise activity. I need the right movement at the right time in the right dose, followed by the right rest. I need enough upright time for essential tasks and enough horizontal time to prevent collapse. I need to spend physical energy only where it matters. A person with limited movement cannot afford waste.

This is the origin of my time management.

People often think of time management as a productivity technique: lists, calendars, priorities, blocks, reminders, efficiency. For me, it is bodily survival. Time is measured not by the clock alone but by tolerance. Fifteen minutes at the sink. Fifteen minutes at the stove. Fifteen minutes unpacking groceries. Fifteen minutes finding a document. Fifteen minutes standing in front of shelves at the press. Fifteen minutes before pain changes the terms.

The body edits the day.

That phrase has become increasingly true. The body cuts, rearranges, deletes, insists, shortens, forbids and occasionally permits. It tells me which ambitions are realistic and which must be translated into another form. If I cannot sit at a desk, I work lying down. If I cannot stand in the kitchen long enough to cook as I once did, I prepare in stages. If I cannot attend an event, I write instead. If I cannot walk far, I organise the room so that what I need is within reach. If I cannot do the whole task, I do the part that matters.

Editing is not failure. Editing is form.

This is perhaps one advantage in the disadvantage. Bertolotti Syndrome has made me ruthless about form. A book must have structure. A meal must have sequence. A painting must have composition. A legal argument must have logic. A day with pain must have architecture. Without structure, everything leaks: time, energy, money, attention, hope.

I have leaked enough.

Sovereign Health is therefore part medicine, part discipline, part defiance and part housekeeping. It is the decision to stop seeking salvation from every new method and start governing the small territory that remains. That territory may be limited, but it is mine. My bed, my desk, my pool, my reformer, my rebounder, my kitchen, my books, my paintings, my press, my legal work, my rules about rest, my cautious use of medication, my refusal to be psychologised again.

There is anger in this, but there is also calm. The anger is for the lost decades. The calm is for the present arrangement. I cannot remake the spine. I can still decide how to live around it.

I can decide that lying down is not defeat.

I can decide that the horizontal life is still a life.

I can decide that the aim is not to impress a doctor with visible activity but to preserve the conditions under which I can write, think, cook, publish, paint and remain recognisably myself.

The medical road may have narrowed. The life has not ended.

10

The Fifteen-Minute Life

The diagnosis changed the story, but it did not change the mechanics of the day.

I still wake up in the same body. The spine has not been remade. The abnormality at the base of the spine remains. The muscles that have spent decades compensating still behave as muscles behave after too much labour, too much guarding, too much collapse and too little structural help. The pain is there before the day has properly formed.

I have become used to beginning from the horizontal.

This is a practical fact before it is a philosophical one. Lying flat is the position in which the body makes the least complaint. It is the position in which I can think, write, read, edit, answer emails, manage a manuscript, organise a publishing task, and sometimes forget the body for long enough to produce something useful. Sitting is often worse than standing. Standing is limited. Walking is difficult. Bending, lifting and twisting have to be rationed. The bed, couch and floor are not places of surrender. They are workstations.

A conventional office assumes a conventional body. A chair, desk, screen, keyboard, meeting room and hour-long conversation all presume that sitting is neutral. For me, sitting is an event. It is something to be planned, monitored and recovered from. A hard chair in a waiting room can change the rest of the day. A café chair can determine how long I can stay with a friend. A meeting can be less demanding intellectually than physically. A desk can be an obstacle disguised as furniture.

So I built another kind of office.

The horizontal office is not elegant. It is efficient. It involves pillows, laptop angles, reading glasses, documents stacked within reach, chargers where they do not require bending, notebooks beside the bed, books arranged so I can access them without unnecessary movement, and a constant awareness of what the body will permit. The room becomes a map of energy. Anything placed too far away may as well be in another country.

This sounds small until one lives it. A pen on the other side of the room. A phone charger under the bed. A book on the floor. A saucepan in a low cupboard. A file in the wrong box. Ordinary objects become tests of planning. A person with a healthy back may reach, bend and retrieve without thinking. I have to ask whether the retrieval is worth the consequence.

My life is organised around these questions.

How many times can I get up? How long can I stand? Which task requires uprightness? Which task can be moved to the bed? Which object should be relocated now so I do not pay for it later? What must be done today, and what only looks urgent because other people organise life around bodies that work differently from mine?

This is how I became a champion time manager.

Time management, in ordinary business language, is about efficiency. It is about calendars, priorities, productivity systems and the conversion of hours into output. My form of time management began before productivity and underneath it. It began with pain. I did not organise time because I wanted to achieve more. I organised time because unorganised time damaged me.

A day has to be designed before it is entered.

There are tasks that can be done lying down: writing, editing, reading, research, emails, planning, website decisions, publishing correspondence, some accounts, manuscript notes, legal thinking, footnote checking, cover comments, poetry drafting, sketching ideas, and the endless administrative work of a small press. There are tasks that must be done upright: showering, dressing, cooking, washing dishes, opening boxes, carrying books, watering plants, dealing with groceries, leaving the house, attending appointments, swimming, reformer work, and the stubborn business of being embodied.

The upright tasks are the expensive ones.

Standing at the sink is one of the worst. The sink is ordinary to most people. It is almost invisible. It sits in the kitchen as part of the background machinery of domestic life. To me, it is a test of endurance. Washing dishes involves standing, bending slightly forward, holding the arms in front of the body, twisting to place objects aside, reaching for cups, shifting weight, and pretending for a few minutes that the spine does not object to any of this.

After a short time, the body begins its argument.

The stove is similar, although more rewarding. Cooking asks for standing, chopping, lifting, stirring and attention. It also gives back colour, smell, taste and hospitality. That makes the calculation different. I will not stand at the sink longer than necessary, but I will spend my limited upright time cooking something that matters. Cooking is not merely feeding myself. It is one of the ways I refuse reduction. A good meal says that life still has form.

The trick is preparation. The task before the task. Vegetables can be washed earlier. Ingredients can be placed on the bench in one trip. Some chopping can be done sitting down. Heavy pots must be avoided or moved with care. A dish that once seemed simple may now be divided into stages. The meal is not made in one burst. It is assembled across the tolerances of the body.

This method has entered everything.

Writing happens in the same way. A book is too large if considered as a single object. A chapter is sometimes too large. A page may be manageable. A paragraph may be enough. A sentence may carry the day. When people see a finished book, they see a whole. I see the fragments: a paragraph written lying flat, a correction made between rests, an email answered before the pain rose, a proof checked in short bursts, a manuscript returned because the body allowed enough concentration that day.

The press runs on fragments.

Clear Mind Press may appear from the outside to be a publishing house, and it is. From the inside, it is also a time-management system. Manuscripts, files, covers, proofs, ISBNs, author emails, printers, distribution channels, sales pages, metadata, errors, corrections, invoices and conversations all have to pass through a body that cannot reliably sit at a desk. Publishing is practical. It is full of small decisions. Small decisions suit a fragmented day if they are organised properly. One can approve a cover lying down. One can edit a paragraph lying down. One can solve a distribution problem lying down. One can build a press from the bed, provided one abandons the fantasy that work must look conventional to be real.

Legal scholarship is different in tone, but similar in method. It requires sustained thought, attention to structure, evidence, citation, argument and consequence. The body interrupts this kind of work constantly, yet the work itself is compatible with stillness. A legal argument can be built in fragments. A difficult idea can be held in the mind while the body rests. A footnote can be checked in a short window. A chapter can be revised across many small sessions. The mind can continue where the spine refuses.

This is why lying down has become central to my intellectual life. It gives me access to the one form of movement the body cannot prevent: thought.

People often misunderstand this. They see the restriction and imagine passivity. They think lying down means doing little. For me, lying down is the condition under which much of the work becomes possible. It is the position from which I have written, edited, studied, organised and published. The horizontal life is not empty. It is densely arranged.

There is discipline in it, but there is also grief.

I would like to stand without calculation. I would like to sit at a table for a whole dinner without assessing the chair. I would like to cook a complicated meal without dividing it into tactical phases. I would like to walk through a gallery slowly, not as a negotiation with pain. I would like to travel without studying the distance from the car park to the door. I would like to go to a café and think only about the friend, the coffee and the conversation. I would like to carry a stack of books without planning the route like a military exercise.

Instead, I measure.

Two hours in a café is the absolute maximum. Often it is too much. I need to know where I can sit, whether I can stand for a moment, whether there is a place to lean, whether I can get back to the car, whether I have enough energy left for the rest of the day. Social life becomes mathematical. That can be painful in a way people do not always see. The restriction is not only physical. It affects spontaneity. It reduces the casual. It turns friendship into planning.

Good friends understand this. They do not take it personally when I leave. They do not require performance. They understand that I may be articulate and in pain at the same time. They understand that conversation can continue while I lie down. They understand that fatigue is not boredom, and departure is not rejection.

Bad systems rarely understand what good friends understand immediately.

The day is held together by routine. Swimming, when I can manage it. The Pilates reformer. The rebounder. Rest. Work. Rest again. A meal. Short bursts of upright activity. More rest. This does not make the pain disappear. It keeps the life possible.

Swimming is the most generous part of the regime. Water changes the terms. In the pool, gravity loosens its grip. The body can move with less argument. I can feel muscles working without the same immediate punishment. It is not a cure. It is a reprieve. Reprieves are valuable.

The reformer gives structure. It helps maintain strength without the chaos of free movement. The rebounder keeps some mobility and circulation alive. These devices sit in my living room like strange domestic companions. They are part gym, part medical equipment, part evidence of persistence. They do not solve the pain. They help me remain someone who can still move.

Rest is the least respected part of the system and the most necessary.

People often treat rest as the opposite of work. For me, rest is the foundation of work. Rest is not what happens after I have finished. It is what makes finishing possible. If I do not rest, I lose the next window. If I lose the next window, the day contracts. If the day contracts too much, the work disappears, the meal disappears, the conversation disappears, and the pain takes more territory.

Rest is infrastructure.

This was one of the hardest lessons to learn because I come from a life of doing. I am not naturally passive. I like making things. Books, poems, paintings, meals, essays, arguments, publishing systems, legal structures. I like the world shaped by intention. Rest can feel like humiliation when the mind is still moving and the body refuses to follow. Yet unmanaged effort is more humiliating. It ends in collapse.

So I rest as a matter of governance.

The fifteen-minute life is not a small life, though it can look small from the outside. It is a life under strict conditions. That is different. A small window can still contain serious work. A short burst can produce a paragraph, a corrected page, a good sauce, a resolved problem, a poem line, an invoice sent, a painting adjusted, a legal idea clarified. The key is not to despise the fragment.

Fragments are how the life is built.

This has changed my understanding of achievement. I no longer believe that significant work requires uninterrupted expanses of time. Expanses are useful, and I would take them if they were available. In their absence, concentration becomes more precise. The question is always: what is the essential action in this window? What has to be done while I am upright? What can wait until I am flat? What will matter tomorrow? What can be abandoned without consequence?

Pain has made me ruthless about unnecessary effort.

That ruthlessness can look severe. It is actually protective. I no longer have enough bodily tolerance for vague obligation. I cannot spend energy on social performance, inefficient systems, badly organised tasks or other people's refusal to understand limits. I need directness. I need clarity. I need the route to be shorter, the chair to be suitable, the task to be real, the meeting to have purpose, the object to be within reach.

In this sense, Bertolotti Syndrome has made me an editor of life. It cuts excess. It marks repetition. It removes decorative difficulty. It asks, again and again: what is the point of this?

That habit serves writing. It serves publishing. It serves scholarship. It serves cooking. It serves survival.

The disadvantage is obvious. Pain, fatigue, weakness, reduced mobility, dependence on planning, loss of spontaneity, a life conducted from the horizontal. The advantage is less obvious, but real. I have become precise. I have learned to distinguish usefulness from noise. I have learned that ten concentrated minutes may be worth more than three vague hours. I have learned that the mind can create continuity even when the body lives in fragments.

This is not triumph. It is design.

I still resent the condition. I resent what was missed. I resent the cost. I resent the years spent trying to fix the wrong problem. I resent the way ordinary tasks have become negotiations. I resent the fact that a sink can defeat me. I resent the hard chair, the long queue, the low cupboard, the heavy box, the cheerful invitation that assumes a body I do not have.

I also know how to work around almost all of it.

That is the strange arithmetic of the fifteen-minute life. The body says no, and the mind asks: in what form can this still be done? Sometimes the answer is that it cannot. More often, the answer is that it can be done differently. Lying down. In stages. With help. With a device. With rest before and after. With fewer movements. With better timing. With less pride. With more precision.

A disadvantage does not automatically contain an advantage. It has to be worked. Sometimes it has to be mined with a pickaxe. Sometimes the advantage is tiny: a better system, a sharper mind, a clearer sentence, a more careful meal, a friend who understands, a morning swim, a paragraph completed before the pain rises.

Tiny advantages count.

They are what remain after the large things have been taken.

11

The Writer Who Changed Languages

Pain has a way of making the body seem like the main character.

It is loud, repetitive and demanding. It interrupts thought. It enters the room before the person does. It shapes the chair, the hour, the journey, the meal, the social invitation, the day's plan and the night's sleep. If one is not careful, pain becomes not only the condition of life but also the subject of it.

I have resisted that.

I was not only a patient. I was a writer long before I had the correct medical word for my pain. I wrote in Dutch before I wrote in English. I wrote fiction, children's books, essays, poems, legal work, reflections on ageing, justice, art and the strange distortions of modern culture. I wrote because language is one of the ways a person refuses to disappear.

The body may narrow movement, but language does not obey the same geography.

I began my writing career in the Netherlands. That was the language in which my early books arrived. Dutch was the language of childhood, memory, streets, shops, weather, irritation, humour, precision and domestic life. It was also the language in which I first learned the professional world of publishing: manuscripts, editors, houses, rejection, acceptance, deadlines, covers, contracts and the strange moment when private sentences become public objects.

There is something bodily about the first language. It sits close to the skin. It knows the family's rhythms, the old jokes, the small humiliations, the childhood rooms. Writing in Dutch was not merely using a vocabulary. It was drawing from the original furniture of the mind.

My first books appeared through established Dutch publishers. I published with Bert Bakker, Atlas and Leopold. This matters because it places my writing life outside the category of hobby. I was not merely someone in pain who kept a journal. I was a professional writer, and my books entered the ordinary world of readers, publishers and translations.

Then came the novel that would travel further than I expected: *De Vismoorden*, later *The Fish Murders*. It was translated into German, French and Spanish before it finally appeared in English. A book can have a more mobile body than its author. It can cross borders without pain, sit on shelves in countries the writer cannot visit, speak in languages the writer did not write, and become part of other people's reading lives. In that sense, publication has always seemed to me a form of escape from the limits of the body.

The body stays. The book travels.

This is perhaps one reason I have always cared so much about publishing. A book is an object that survives the hour of its making. It allows fragmented work to become whole. It turns short bursts of effort into something with a spine of its own. That metaphor is almost too obvious for me, but it is unavoidable. My spine has failed me in many ways; my books have carried themselves upright.

The writer's life, however, was never separate from pain. I did not write in a clean, protected room away from the body. I wrote inside the body I had. I wrote around children, work, migration, relationships, anxiety, treatment, medical appointments and fatigue. I wrote in the gaps. I wrote when I could sit, and later when I could not. I wrote through uncertainty. I wrote even when my back made the ordinary arrangements of literary life difficult.

People often imagine writing as a sedentary occupation and therefore physically easy. It is not. Sitting is an act. A chair is a proposition. A desk is a demand. A long writing session assumes that the body can remain still without becoming the main problem. Mine could not. Even before I understood this fully, I was already finding ways to write in fragments, to return to the page after interruption, to carry a sentence through pain, to stop before collapse, and to resume later as if the broken line were continuous.

Writing taught me continuity under interruption.

That lesson would later become central to the fifteen-minute life. A manuscript is not written in one heroic stretch. It is made by returning. Pain interrupts, children interrupt, work interrupts, migration interrupts, life interrupts, but the page permits return. A paragraph can wait. A character can wait. An idea can wait. The writer's task is to keep the thread alive.

For many years, I kept that thread in Dutch.

Then I moved to Australia.

Changing countries is difficult enough. Changing writing language is a deeper kind of migration. Speaking a language and writing literature in it are not the same thing. A person can live in English, shop in English, work in English, argue in English and dream occasionally in English, yet still not possess the full range of literary instinct. Writing requires more than correctness. It requires rhythm, humour, register, nerve and the ability to hear when a sentence is false.

It took years to make the change.

In the beginning, English felt like a room with furniture placed slightly wrongly. I could move through it, but I bumped into things.

Some words were too formal, some too flat, some too emotional, some not quite mine. Dutch remained the earlier room, familiar but increasingly distant from the life I was living. I had to decide whether to remain a Dutch writer living elsewhere or become an English-language writer with a Dutch past.

The body, meanwhile, had its own opinions. Pain does not wait politely while a person changes language. It continued to require management. It continued to interrupt. The work of linguistic migration had to be done inside the same constrained body that had already carried me through Europe, Japan and Australia.

There is an advantage, perhaps, in having lived across languages with a body that never allowed complacency. I had already learned not to assume that ease was available. English became another discipline, another set of muscles, another asymmetry to work with. One side of the mind moved easily; the other had to be trained. The metaphor was familiar.

Over time, English became not only the language I lived in, but the language I wrote in. The shift changed the work. It made the sentences cleaner in some ways, stranger in others. It gave me distance from the old self. It also gave me access to the country in which I was now living, thinking and arguing. Australia became not simply a place of residence but a language of work.

I wrote *The Elephant's Tooth*. I wrote about crime in Alice Springs and rural Australia. I wrote about justice, old age, art, ikigai, artificial intelligence and kitsch. I wrote poems. I wrote short essays on drawing, seeing and looking. I wrote because the mind, once trained to move, does not accept confinement easily.

Poetry deserves its own place in this story.

A poem is a small form with large pressure. It suits a fragmented life because it can be held in the mind in pieces. A line can arrive when the body is resting. A rhythm can develop while the back is bad. A sonnet, especially, imposes a discipline that pain understands. It has limits. It has structure. It has a shape that must be honoured. The sonnet does not say: express everything. It says: work inside this frame.

I know something about frames.

Pain is a frame. Language is a frame. Law is a frame. A book is a frame. A body is a frame. The question is never whether there are limits. There are always limits. The question is what can still be made inside them.

That is why writing and Bertolotti Syndrome cannot be separated in this book. The condition did not make me a writer. I reject that kind of sentimental causation. I did not need pain in order to have a mind. But pain changed the methods by which the writing happened. It made me economical. It made me intolerant of waste. It made me sharp about structure. It made me think in units. It made me ask what mattered in a paragraph, a chapter, a book and a day.

Writing also gave me a way not to be consumed by the medical story. Each book said: the pain is here, but it is not the only thing here. Each manuscript extended the self beyond the body's immediate complaint. Each completed work proved that a restricted body could still produce an unrestricted intellectual life.

This is not the same as optimism. It is evidence.

There are many kinds of evidence in a life. Medical imaging is one kind. Blood tests, scans, diagnoses and clinical notes are others. But books are also evidence. Poems are evidence. Paintings are evidence. Meals are evidence. A publishing house is evidence. They show that the life was not empty, even when the body was difficult. They show that the person was not reducible to the symptom.

For years, doctors failed to see my body properly. There is a strange parallel in the way people sometimes fail to see a disabled or chronically ill person's work properly. If the work exists, they minimise the illness. If the illness is emphasised, they minimise the work. They find it difficult to hold both together: severe physical constraint and serious productivity; daily pain and humour; lying down and running a press; needing a walking stick and writing legal scholarship; being unable to stand at the sink and still cooking beautifully.

But both are true.

The truth is not balanced by softening either side. The pain is severe. The work is real. The body is restricted. The life is large. The diagnosis came too late. The books still exist.

This is one reason I want this book to hold the whole story. The medical narrative alone would make me disappear into pathology. The literary narrative alone would make the pain look like a footnote. Neither version is true. The truth is that I wrote through the whole thing, sometimes because of discipline, sometimes because of fury, sometimes because writing was the only place left where I could move without asking permission.

Writing is a place where no doctor can tell me to sit down.

It is also a place where the misdiagnosis can be answered. Not cured, not reversed, but answered. The unanswered pain of the body becomes language. The scattered decades become chapters. The wrong explanations become part of a pattern. The invisible becomes visible. The patient becomes narrator.

That matters more than I once understood.

A patient is usually spoken about. The doctor writes the notes. The report interprets the image. The specialist gives the opinion. The pharmacist labels the bottle. The system creates the file. In writing, the direction reverses. I describe the body. I arrange the evidence. I choose the frame. I decide what matters. I say what was missed.

The page gives back jurisdiction.

Perhaps that is why I kept writing across languages, countries and diagnoses. Writing was never simply expression. It was governance. It was a way to make order where other systems had produced confusion. It was a way to carry the self from Dutch into English, from Europe into Australia, from pain into thought, from private endurance into public form.

The writer who changed languages did not leave the old body behind. She brought it with her. She wrote from it, around it, against it and sometimes because it forced her into a chair, then out of the chair, then onto the bed, where the next sentence was still waiting.

12

The Law Is Equally Narrow-Minded

Law entered my life as another way of asking what systems see and what they miss.

By then, I had spent decades inside medical systems that looked authoritative from the outside and inadequate from the inside. I had been examined, scanned, adjusted, medicated, reassured, doubted, psychologised and redirected. The body had been handled by many professions, but the actual structure causing the trouble had remained unnamed. A small abnormality at the base of the spine had shaped a whole life while remaining outside the frame of attention.

That experience changes the way a person thinks.

It made me suspicious of categories that arrive too quickly. It made me attentive to the difference between evidence and interpretation. It made me aware that a system can be procedurally correct and substantively wrong. A doctor can order the scan, read the report, follow the usual pathway and still fail to understand the patient. The problem is not always absence of process. Sometimes the problem is the narrowness of the process itself.

Law has its own forms of narrowness.

A legal system must classify. It must sort events, persons, harms, claims, duties and remedies into forms that can be handled. Without classification, law cannot function. Yet the same classificatory impulse can produce injustice when the category becomes stronger than the reality it is meant to serve. A person becomes a complainant, defendant, offender, victim, applicant, tenant, patient, child, creditor, debtor or risk. The legal file begins to stand in for the life.

This was familiar to me.

Medicine had already placed me under inadequate headings: leg-length discrepancy, muscular pain, myofascial pain, anxiety, wear and tear, TMS, non-specific back pain. Each category contained a fragment of plausibility. None contained the truth. The labels were harmful because they reduced inquiry. Once a person has been assigned to the wrong category, the system may continue to operate with confidence while moving further away from reality.

In law, I saw the same danger at a different scale.

The law is skilled at looking where it has been trained to look. It can be precise, technical, disciplined and powerful. It can also be dangerously partial. It may attend to one actor and ignore the system around that actor. It may punish an individual while overlooking the social, economic, environmental or institutional conditions that shaped the event. It may protect procedure while failing to produce justice. It may speak in the language of rights and duties while avoiding the deeper question of whether the arrangement itself is sustainable.

This is where my work on Sustainable Justice began to matter to me in a deeply personal way.

I did not set out to turn back pain into jurisprudence. That would be too neat and too self-serving. My thesis was not a memoir in disguise. Yet no serious intellectual project is entirely separate from the life of the person who pursues it. We choose questions partly because they have already chosen us. My body had taught me, long before I entered legal scholarship, that systems can fail by looking too narrowly. It had taught me that suffering often occurs in the gap between lived reality and institutional recognition. It had taught me that the wrong frame can become a source of harm.

The phrase that joined these worlds came after my diagnosis.

I told my supervisors about Bertolotti Syndrome. I explained that, for forty-eight years, doctors had looked at my spine and had not looked three centimetres to the right of it. One of my supervisors said, "This is exactly what your thesis is about. The law is equally narrow-minded."

That sentence clarified something I had already known but had not fully articulated.

Three centimetres to the right became more than an anatomical location. It became a metaphor for institutional failure. The relevant evidence may be close. It may be visible. It may sit beside the recognised object of attention. Yet if the system has not been trained to assign significance to it, it disappears. The scan exists, but the diagnosis does not. The person speaks, but the system hears only what its categories permit. The harm is present, but the remedy is elsewhere.

In medicine, this produced decades of misdiagnosis. In law, it can produce whole patterns of injustice.

A narrow legal system may ask whether a rule has been breached while failing to ask whether the rule itself is adequate. It may ask whether a person has chosen freely while ignoring constraints that make meaningful choice doubtful. It may ask whether harm can be proved within an existing evidentiary frame while ignoring harms that accumulate slowly, collectively or intergenerationally. It may ask whether a procedure was followed while ignoring whether the procedure was capable of producing a just result.

These are not abstract concerns. Systems organise consequences. If the frame is wrong, the consequences can be wrong even when the internal logic is tidy.

Chronic pain trained me to understand this at the level of the body. If a doctor assumes the pain is muscular, the treatment will be muscular. If the doctor assumes the pain is psychological, the patient will be directed towards the mind. If the doctor assumes the abnormal vertebra is incidental, the relevant structure will not be investigated. Each assumption produces a pathway. Each pathway consumes time, money, hope and bodily capacity. The wrong frame is not intellectually neutral. It has material effects.

Legal frames have material effects too.

This is why I became interested in justice as something larger than a court outcome. A system can deliver a formally correct result and still leave the underlying conditions untouched. It can process cases while reproducing the patterns that generated them. It can protect rights on paper while leaving people without the practical conditions in which those rights can be exercised. It can focus on immediate actors while ignoring future consequences. It can treat the environment, future generations, non-human life, communities and vulnerable people as peripheral because the traditional frame has been built around narrower subjects.

Sustainable Justice, as I developed it, was my attempt to think beyond that narrowness.

The concept required me to consider justice through systems, relationships, time and consequence. It asked how legal and institutional arrangements might become more responsive to interconnected forms of harm. It asked how justice might be evaluated when the effects of decisions extend beyond the immediate parties, beyond the courtroom, beyond the present generation and beyond human convenience. It required attention to context, complexity and responsibility.

These questions were intellectually demanding. They were also bodily familiar.

I knew what it meant to live inside a system that treated the immediate presentation as the whole problem. I knew what it meant to have the wrong evidence privileged and the right evidence ignored. I knew what it meant for an explanation to be plausible enough to delay the truth. I knew what it meant for a person to become exhausted by institutions that require repetition of the same story without producing learning. I knew what it meant to pay for other people's narrowness.

The body had already given me the method: look wider.

Legal scholarship gave that method language.

It also gave structure to a life that might otherwise have been reduced to management of symptoms. A PhD is not a small undertaking, even for a person without chronic pain. It requires years of reading, thinking, drafting, revising, defending, doubting and returning. It asks the mind to hold a large argument over a long period of time. It is both intellectual work and endurance work.

For me, it was also physical work.

The thesis was written in fragments, often while lying down. The body set the conditions. I could not simply sit at a desk for hours like the fantasy scholar of old libraries and wooden chairs. I had to build the argument around pain. Reading required posture. Writing required arrangement. Footnotes required concentration. Revisions required stamina. Supervisor comments had to be absorbed on days when the body had already used much of its capacity getting through ordinary life.

Yet scholarship suited the horizontal life. It required stillness, and I had plenty of enforced stillness. It required attention, and pain had trained attention brutally. It required patience with complexity, and my life had long since destroyed any appetite for simple answers. It required resistance to premature closure, and misdiagnosis had made me distrust closure that arrived too easily.

The thesis became another form of movement.

This is difficult to explain to people who identify movement only with the body. Intellectual work moves differently. It travels through texts, arguments, histories, cases, theories and systems. It moves from a question to a method, from method to structure, from structure to claim, from claim to revision. It crosses disciplines. It brings one idea into relation with another. For a person whose body is increasingly restricted, this kind of movement is not secondary. It is a form of freedom.

That freedom was never romantic. It was hard, often tedious, frequently painful and sometimes absurd. A body that cannot stand at a sink for long can still spend hours wrestling with a paragraph about justice. That is both comic and serious. It shows the mismatch between bodily incapacity and intellectual stamina. It also shows why disability cannot be understood through outward function alone.

I was, by many ordinary measures, highly functional. I could write a thesis. I could run arguments. I could read difficult material. I could hold an idea across years. I could publish books. Yet I could not sit comfortably, stand reliably, walk easily, clean without help, garden without help, or cook without planning. This combination confused people. It still does.

Law should understand such combinations better than it often does. Disability, capacity, responsibility, vulnerability and agency are rarely simple. A person may be capable in one domain and severely limited in another. A person may have strong intellect and weak mobility. A person may be productive because she has built severe systems around herself, not because the condition is mild. A person may appear articulate in the very moment she is physically close to collapse.

The legal imagination often struggles with these mixed states. So does medicine. So does ordinary social life.

My work on Sustainable Justice made me ask what a more adequate system would need. It would need to attend to complexity without becoming paralysed by it. It would need to hold individual agency and structural conditions together. It would need to recognise that harms can be distributed across time, systems and bodies. It would need to treat lived experience as evidence without abandoning critical reasoning. It would need to ask what has been left just outside the frame.

Three centimetres to the right.

That phrase still matters because it is concrete. It prevents abstraction from floating away. The missed structure was not somewhere mystical or inaccessible. It was close. It was visible to the right kind of attention. It had been there from the beginning. The failure was interpretive.

A legal scholar learns that interpretation is never innocent.

Facts do not simply speak. They are selected, weighed, classified and connected. Evidence is made legally meaningful through frames. The same is true in medicine. A transitional vertebra may be seen and dismissed as incidental, or seen and understood as clinically significant. A patient's anxiety may be treated as the cause of pain, or as evidence of what untreated pain has done. A scan may be read as normal because the reader is looking for the usual problem. A life may be misread because the person appears too competent to be suffering as much as she says.

This is why justice requires humility.

Certainty is attractive to systems. It speeds decisions. It reassures professionals. It reduces complexity. It allows a file to move. Yet premature certainty can be a form of violence. It tells the patient, litigant, tenant, complainant, prisoner, student or citizen that the system has finished seeing before the person has finished being understood.

I had been on the receiving end of that many times.

The PhD did not take away the pain, but it gave me a larger framework in which to understand it. My body was not only a private misfortune. It was also a case study in institutional limitation: what happens when a system has insufficient categories for a real condition; what happens when experiential evidence is discounted; what happens when delay becomes harm; what happens when a person pays for professional ignorance over decades; what happens when the wrong explanation becomes a life.

The scholarly task was to think beyond the personal without abandoning what the personal had taught.

That is the balance I have tried to keep. A memoir can become too private. A thesis can become too abstract. Life requires movement between the two. My back gave me material I would never have chosen. Law gave me a language that could place individual suffering inside wider patterns. Publishing gave me a way to send those patterns into the world.

By the time my diagnosis arrived, I was in the last phase of the thesis. This timing felt almost too precise. After decades of bodily misrecognition, the name of the condition appeared just as I was completing a major work about broader justice, systems and the need to see beyond inherited frames. It did not make the pain meaningful in any easy sense. Pain does not need to be redeemed to be understood. But it did reveal a continuity between the body and the work.

I had been studying narrowness all along.

The law is equally narrow-minded. The sentence was true, but it was also a challenge. If law is narrow, it can be widened. If medicine is narrow, it can be taught to look differently. If a scan can be misread, a person can insist on another reading. If a system has failed, the failure can be documented. If a life has been misclassified, it can be narrated again, this time from the inside.

This book belongs to that work.

It is not a legal thesis. It is not a medical textbook. It is the account of a life in which the same lesson kept appearing in different forms: look properly; listen carefully; do not let the category replace the person; do not assume that what has not been named is not real; do not mistake confidence for knowledge; do not build systems that function by ignoring the evidence they were not trained to value.

A good legal system, like a good doctor, must know how to look three centimetres to the right.

13

The Publishing House from the Bed

Clear Mind Press began as an act of independence.

That is the simplest way to say it. It was not born from a corporate strategy, a marketing plan, a grant, a committee, or a desire to build a large publishing machine. It began because I wanted to publish work that did not fit neatly into the available channels, and because I had reached a point in life where I no longer wanted permission from institutions that had shown themselves too often to be timid, fashionable, bureaucratic or narrow.

Publishing is, in that sense, a form of jurisdiction. It decides what enters public form. It takes a manuscript, which may have existed for years as a private labour, and gives it a cover, page numbers, ISBN, metadata, distribution pathway, price, description, category and visible place in the world. Publishing is not only printing. It is the conversion of thought into an object that can travel.

I have always liked that about books.

Books have bodies, but they are not trapped in mine. They move where I cannot move. They sit upright on shelves. They are mailed across distances. They arrive in houses, libraries, bookshops and waiting rooms. They enter conversations without asking whether I can stand, sit or walk that day. A book can go to a reader while I am lying down with my spine refusing the most ordinary forms of movement.

There is a kind of justice in that.

Clear Mind Press was established in 2022, first to publish *The Elephant's Tooth*. That book belonged to my work on crime, justice and rural Australia, and it needed a publisher with enough courage and practical flexibility to take it on. I did not want to wait for permission. I did not want to reshape the work to please a commercial gatekeeper. I did not want the material softened into something safer or more fashionable. So I made the publishing house myself.

This sounds grander than it was. In practice, founding a small press means learning a thousand unglamorous tasks. ISBNs. Covers. Copyright pages. Editing. Proofreading. Metadata. Distribution. Print specifications. ePub conversion. File sizes. Trim sizes. Margins. Fonts. Invoices. Emails. Stock. Bookshops. Websites. Author anxieties. Printer errors. Price points. Blurbs. Back matter. Indexing. Permissions. Rights. Sales reports. Delivery failures. Corrections that appear only after the proof has supposedly been finalised.

Publishing is full of small mistakes waiting to happen.

That suited me more than I expected. A person who lives with chronic pain becomes accustomed to managing detail because detail is where the day succeeds or fails. The difference between an object placed within reach and one placed on the floor can determine whether a task is simple or painful. The difference between a chair and a couch can determine whether a meeting is possible. The difference between doing something now and doing it in ten minutes can determine whether the rest of the day collapses.

A small press is also made of such differences.

A comma in the wrong place. A cover image at the wrong resolution. A file named incorrectly. A paragraph repeated. A page number missing.

A typo in a title. A printer's template misunderstood. A distribution field left blank. A contributor's name misspelt. None of these things is dramatic in itself. Together, they decide whether a book appears professional or careless.

Pain had made me impatient with carelessness.

This is one of the unexpected advantages in the disadvantage. Bertolotti Syndrome did not make me a publisher, but it trained some of the habits publishing requires: attention, sequencing, stamina in fragments, suspicion of vague promises, the ability to return to a problem after interruption, and a fairly ruthless distinction between what matters and what merely makes noise.

I could not work like a conventional publisher in a conventional office. I could not sit at a desk all day with a pile of manuscripts and a clear calendar. I could not attend every event, drive to every meeting, stand behind a table at every book fair, or carry boxes of stock as if books were weightless because they belonged to the life of the mind.

Books are not weightless. A carton of books is an argument with the spine.

So the press had to be built around my body. The bed became part of the office. The couch became part of the office. The laptop became a printing press in miniature. The email inbox became a loading dock. A publishing decision could be made lying flat with a hot pack, a manuscript, and a cup of tea within reach. A book could be edited in short windows. A cover could be considered from the horizontal. An author could be reassured from the bed. A problem with a file could be solved between pain flares.

This did not make the work less real. It made the work more exact.

The title "Clear Mind Press" mattered to me. I wanted clarity. I wanted independence. I wanted books that carried human voices, not formulaic products assembled to satisfy a market trend. The press described itself as fiercely independent. That was not branding invented by a consultant. It was a position. I had become suspicious of sleepy institutions and equally suspicious of ideological conformity dressed as virtue. I wanted to publish work that was awake to the present without becoming obedient to fashion.

The same instinct had been sharpened by the body.

A person who has spent decades being told the wrong thing becomes less impressed by consensus. Consensus can be useful. It can also be lazy. Many people agreed, implicitly or explicitly, that my back pain was muscular, postural, psychological, ordinary, stress-related, or a matter of wear and tear. They were not correct because they agreed with one another. They were simply wrong in similar ways.

Publishing requires a related independence. The question is not always whether a manuscript fits what is currently easy to sell. Sometimes the question is whether the manuscript contains a human necessity that should exist in public form. That is why small presses matter. They can publish from conviction rather than only from predicted scale.

Of course conviction does not remove the practical burden. A small press still has to pay for editing, design, production, distribution and mistakes. It still has to think about readers. It still has to make the book work in the world. Independence without competence is indulgence. I did not want indulgence. I wanted books that were carefully made.

This is where my life as editor, writer and legal scholar entered the press. Editing requires respect for the author's voice, but also firmness. A manuscript is not improved by drowning it in someone else's style. It is improved by finding its own spine. That metaphor returns again. A book needs a spine. It needs structure strong enough to carry the material. If the structure is weak, the book collapses under its own intention.

I knew something about collapse.

The Bertolotti Syndrome book was one of the most demanding publishing projects I had undertaken. It required the coordination of personal stories, medical information, academic articles, patient resources, disclaimers, permissions, terminology, diagrams, and the emotional reality of people who had been dismissed for years. It had to be clear enough for patients and serious enough for doctors. It had to hold anger without becoming incoherent. It had to give patients a voice without pretending that personal experience alone could replace medical reasoning.

That balance mattered.

People living with Bertolotti Syndrome often arrive with rage, and the rage is understandable. Years or decades of dismissal do not produce polite gratitude. They produce frustration, grief, suspicion and sometimes fury. Yet a book addressed also to doctors cannot simply shout. It has to persuade. It has to document. It has to distinguish what is known, what is probable, what is contested and what is only lived experience. The task was to preserve the force of patient testimony while maintaining enough clarity and discipline for the book to be useful.

That is publishing as justice work.

It is also exhausting work. The body did not stop hurting because the project mattered. If anything, important projects are more dangerous because they tempt me to override the body. A deadline, an author waiting, a proof arriving, a printer problem, a chapter needing revision: these things create urgency. Urgency is the enemy of a body with Bertolotti Syndrome. It encourages standing too long, sitting too long, concentrating beyond the body's tolerance, skipping rest, pushing through, and paying later.

I have paid later many times.

Still, publishing gave me something pain could not take easily: purpose structured into tasks. A press creates external obligations. Authors need answers. Readers need books. Files need correction. Projects need finishing. This can be burdensome, but it can also be protective. Pain narrows the world inward. Work sends attention outward. Editing another person's manuscript moves the mind away from the body's complaint and towards a text that needs care.

That outward movement is valuable.

It is one reason I have never accepted the idea that rest and work are opposites. The press exists because I rest enough to work and work carefully enough to justify rest. The horizontal office is not a retreat from public life. It is the condition under which I can remain in it.

There is also a social dimension to publishing that suited the restricted life. A press gathers people without requiring all of them to be physically present. Authors, editors, designers, proofreaders, readers and printers can form a working community through manuscripts and files. For someone whose mobility is limited, that matters. The work can be relational without requiring constant physical attendance. It allows connection through books.

The Bertolotti book made this especially clear. I spoke with people living with the condition. Their stories varied enormously, but certain patterns returned: delayed diagnosis, disbelief, pain, fatigue, high-functioning minds inside limited bodies, and a need for careful time management. I recognised myself in them, and they recognised something in one another. The book became more than a publication. It became a gathering point for people whose condition had often made them isolated.

A small press can do that. It can make a room where no room existed.

From the outside, the work may look like administration. From the inside, it is an attempt to give form to voices that might otherwise remain scattered. A personal story becomes a chapter. A chapter becomes part of a book. A book becomes a resource. A resource enters a consultation room, a support group, a family conversation, perhaps even a doctor's education. That is not abstract. It is practical.

I have often thought that books are among the most efficient devices humans have made for transferring attention. A book says: look here, and keep looking. It slows the reader down. It arranges evidence. It preserves memory. It allows a person who may not be physically present to insist on being heard.

For a woman living much of her life lying down, that matters deeply.

Clear Mind Press also allowed me to bring the different parts of myself under one roof. The writer, editor, publisher, legal scholar, poet and painter did not have to compete for separate legitimacy. They could all serve the making of books. The legal scholar cared about argument, fairness, evidence and systems. The writer cared about language. The poet cared about compression. The painter cared about form and seeing. The cook cared about sequence, timing and presentation. The patient cared about the body, the cost of being unheard, and the need to respect lived experience without surrendering to confusion.

All of those selves were useful in publishing.

Cooking and publishing are more alike than they appear. Both require preparation, timing, order and judgement. Both require knowing when something is overdone, underdone, too heavy, too thin, too cluttered or not yet coherent. Both involve serving something to others. Both can be ruined by haste. Both reward attention to small details that inexperienced people think are trivial.

Painting and publishing also belong together. A cover is not decoration. It is the book's first argument about itself. White space matters. Line matters. Balance matters. The eye understands things before the mind has named them. A poorly made book can undermine its own content before the first sentence is read. A carefully made book invites trust.

Poetry, too, has its place in the press. A publisher must understand compression. A blurb is a small form with disproportionate power. A title can make a book visible or bury it. A subtitle can clarify or confuse.

Metadata is prose under commercial pressure. Even a copyright page has its own dry poetics if one has spent enough time with books.

The press became a way of practising all these disciplines under one roof, even when the roof was sometimes simply the ceiling above my bed.

I do not want to make this sound romantic. Running a small press is hard, uncertain and often financially irrational. It requires stubbornness, money, taste, patience and a tolerance for problems that appear at the worst possible time. It also requires a degree of invisibility. Readers see the book. They do not see the hundreds of small decisions that made it possible. They do not see the body lying down between tasks.

But perhaps that is appropriate. Much of a good book should be invisible. The labour should support the reading, not interrupt it. A book is successful when the reader enters the work without constantly seeing the scaffolding. A painful life is similar. If the systems are well designed, others may not see how much work it takes to remain functional.

This invisibility has a cost. People underestimate the effort. They see the finished book and assume the process was manageable. They see the output and assume the body was equal to it. They see productivity and assume health. They are wrong, but understandably wrong. The systems are designed to hide the collapse.

I know this now, and I no longer apologise for it.

The press is one of the clearest examples of the advantage inside the disadvantage. The disadvantage is obvious: I cannot run a publishing house in the ordinary upright, mobile, event-heavy way. The advantage is that limitation forced the press to become precise, lean, independent and intensely text-focused. It forced me to design processes around reality rather than fantasy. It forced me to ask what publishing actually requires, once the theatrical parts are stripped away.

It requires judgement. It requires attention. It requires language. It requires structure. It requires persistence. It requires respect for the reader. It requires respect for the author. It requires the ability to finish.

All of those can be done from a bed.

14

The Kitchen and the Studio

The kitchen is one of the places where pain becomes most visible.

This may sound strange, because kitchens are usually associated with warmth, appetite, family, friendship and domestic competence. Mine has been all of those things. I have always loved cooking. I love the transformation of ingredients into food, the sequence of preparation, the smell of onions softening, the judgement of heat, the timing of several small tasks that have to meet at the right moment. Cooking is one of the arts that does not announce itself too loudly as art. It happens close to necessity. People have to eat. Yet, within that necessity, there is form, style, care, abundance and intelligence.

I have been a good cook for a long time.

That matters because cooking is one of the pleasures Bertolotti Syndrome tried to take from me. It did not take it all at once. Chronic pain rarely removes a life by dramatic seizure. It takes things by making them more costly. First a meal becomes tiring. Then a complicated meal becomes risky. Then the standing has to be broken into sections. Then the saucepan is too heavy. Then the washing up is worse than the cooking. Then shopping becomes part of the calculation. Then one begins to understand that a kitchen is full of small physical demands masquerading as ordinary life.

A kitchen assumes a body that can stand.

It assumes the cook can bend to reach a pan, lift a pot, carry groceries, unload a dishwasher, open a low cupboard, twist towards a drawer, stand over a sink, chop for ten minutes, stir, wash, wipe, turn, reach, taste and remain upright long enough for the meal to come together. It assumes these actions are minor. For me, each of them has a price.

Standing at the sink is nearly impossible now. The position is brutal: slightly forward, arms in front, spine loaded, body locked into a posture that seems harmless until the pain rises. Washing dishes is therefore one of the least poetic tasks in my life. It has none of the reward of cooking and all of the punishment. The sink is where romance about the domestic life ends.

The stove is different. The stove gives back.

I will spend energy on food because food gives something in return. A meal is a form of order. It is evidence that life still has taste, colour, sequence and generosity. It says that the body has limits, but the day has not become purely medical. Pain may dictate how long I can stand, but it does not decide whether a meal can have flavour.

The method has changed. I cook now through strategy. I prepare before I prepare. I bring ingredients to the bench in as few trips as possible. I sit when something can be done sitting down. I choose dishes according to the amount of standing they require, the weight of the pots, the cleaning afterwards, the number of steps between fridge, sink, stove and table. I no longer judge a recipe only by taste. I judge it by its demands on the spine.

There are recipes that are delicious and therefore impossible.

This is the kind of knowledge chronic pain produces. It is precise, unglamorous and rarely visible from the outside. A guest sees the meal. The guest does not see the calculation: what was chopped earlier, what was abandoned, what was bought already prepared, what was cooked in stages, how long I lay down between tasks, what I decided was worth the pain and what was not. Good cooking can hide a great deal.

It is the same with almost everything I do.

The meal appears whole because the fragments have been made to co-operate. The chapter appears whole because the paragraphs were assembled across pain, rest and return. The painting appears whole because the hand found its way across the paper, even if the body could not remain where it wanted to remain. The press appears whole because the emails, proofs, covers and production tasks were handled in small windows. A life can look continuous when it has actually been constructed from interruptions.

Cooking taught me this long before I named it.

A dish is built through sequence. Some things must come first. Some things must wait. Some things can be prepared hours earlier. Some things cannot be rushed. Some ingredients collapse if overhandled. Some flavours need quiet. Some mistakes can be corrected. Others cannot. A person who cooks well learns to think in systems, timings and consequences. This is also how a painful life has to be managed.

The kitchen therefore became both pleasure and training.

It trained attention. It trained order. It trained improvisation. It trained respect for limits. It trained the discipline of doing the necessary thing at the right moment rather than the dramatic thing too late. It also trained the acceptance of compromise. A good meal made under physical constraint may not be the meal one would cook in a younger or stronger body, but it can still be good. It can still carry care.

Care is important.

When pain has been severe for decades, there is a danger that the body becomes a technical problem and the person becomes the technician of that problem. Exercises, appointments, medications, devices, scans, specialists, referrals, pain scores, waiting lists. All of that may be necessary, but none of it is enough. A person also needs beauty, taste, friendship, texture, humour and the ordinary dignity of making something pleasing.

Cooking kept me human in that way.

Painting did the same, though through another route.

Painting does not begin with necessity. It begins with seeing. It asks one to notice shape, negative space, weight, light, proportion, line, gesture, colour and the relationship between what is present and what is missing. In that sense, painting belongs very naturally with a life marked by misdiagnosis. For decades, people looked at me and did not see what mattered. They looked at images and did not interpret them properly. They looked at symptoms and fitted them into inadequate categories. They looked at the person and missed the body.

Painting is a way of looking properly.

It has always interested me that the visual evidence of my condition was present long before the medical name arrived. Photographs show what the clinical encounters failed to register. The asymmetry was there. The lopsidedness was there. Even clothing adjusted itself around the body's shape. In the silhouette photographs included in the Bertolotti book, the body speaks with an almost brutal clarity. The raised, truncated right hip can be seen. The distortion is not an abstract complaint. It is visible.

This is why the silhouettes mattered so much to me.

They were not glamorous images. They were evidence. They said: look. They said: this body has been trying to tell you something. They said: why did nobody notice? They said: do not look only at the computer screen, the report, the standard diagnostic pathway. Look at the person in front of you.

For years, I had felt unseen by doctors. I do not mean emotionally unseen, though that was often true as well. I mean physically unseen. The body itself had not been observed carefully enough. The asymmetry, the way I stood, the way I moved, the way clothes sat on me, the history of stumbling, the one-sidedness in dance, the groin pain, the hip, the back attacks: these were not obscure clues. They required attention.

The silhouettes became my answer to that failure.

They also connected to the painter's mind. A painter understands that a form can be distorted and still coherent. A line can carry tension. A shadow can reveal structure. What is left out can matter as much as what is drawn. The body in silhouette removes distraction. It leaves outline, tilt, proportion and imbalance. It makes visible what ordinary viewing may soften.

There is anger in those images.

There is also discipline.

Anger alone does not make art. It may start the movement, but the image still has to work. It needs form. It needs restraint. It needs enough distance that the viewer can look without being shouted at, while still understanding that something has been missed. This is also true of writing about pain. A howl may be true, but it cannot carry a whole book. The material has to be shaped so that another person can enter it.

This is where my lives as writer, painter, cook, publisher and scholar meet. Each requires form under pressure. Each requires selection. Each refuses the raw condition as the final state. A pile of ingredients is not a meal. A pile of memories is not a book. A pile of evidence is not an argument. A pile of paint is not a painting. A pile of symptoms is not a diagnosis.

Form matters.

Pain, however, is hostile to form. It disrupts. It breaks concentration. It forces cancellations. It collapses sequence. It turns a morning plan into an afternoon recovery. It makes the hand unreliable. It makes the back intolerant. It makes the simplest act require negotiation. It interrupts the gesture before the line is finished. It interrupts the thought before the sentence has settled. It interrupts the meal before the table is cleared.

The work of my life has been to reintroduce form after interruption.

This is why I find comfort in small rituals. Japanese tea ceremony entered my life partly through the aesthetics of Japan and partly through the needs of my present body. My hands are affected now. I drop things. Fine motor control is not always reliable. Offering Japanese tea ceremony to friends became a way to practise the hands without making the practice clinical. It turns rehabilitation into hospitality. It gives clumsy hands something dignified to do.

That is important. I do not want every exercise to look like exercise. I do not want every bodily practice to be medicalised. I have had enough of the medical gaze. A movement can be therapeutic without looking like treatment. A bowl can be lifted with care. A whisk can be held. Water can be poured. A cup can be offered. The hand practises steadiness, but the social meaning is tea.

This is a better arrangement for the soul.

The tea ceremony also suits the fifteen-minute life. It is structured. It has order. It values attention over speed. It accepts that small actions can carry meaning. It does not require grand movement. It requires presence, exactness and respect for the object. Those qualities are compatible with a body that must move carefully.

In tea, as in cooking and painting, there is no separation between practical action and aesthetic judgement. The way something is placed matters. The angle of the hand matters. The surface matters. The timing matters. A small gesture can be crude or graceful. A person living with pain learns this as well. There are crude ways to move through pain and more graceful ways. Grace does not remove pain. It prevents pain from becoming the only visible fact.

I do not always manage grace.

Some days I am irritated, clumsy, impatient and tired. Some days I drop things and swear. Some days the kitchen defeats me. Some days the studio is unreachable. Some days the hands will not co-operate. Some days ready-made food from a café is the sensible choice, and the sensible choice is still disappointing. Some days the only form available is survival.

That, too, belongs in the story.

There is a danger in writing about adaptation that it can make adaptation sound elegant. Much of it is not. Much of it is tedious. It involves fatigue, resentment, mess, small humiliations and the shrinking of ordinary options. I do not want to turn the painful life into an aesthetic lifestyle. Bertolotti Syndrome is not a design principle. It is a disabling condition.

Yet I have had to design around it.

The kitchen had to be redesigned in practice, even when the furniture remained the same. The studio had to become flexible. The office had to become horizontal. The social life had to become timed. The body had to become a calendar. The day had to become a sequence of windows. Within those constraints, I still wanted good food, good books, good lines, good colours, good conversations and good arguments.

That desire has kept me from becoming purely medical.

A person with chronic pain can spend enormous energy proving pain. There are forms, applications, consultations, explanations, sceptical faces, repeated histories, pain scales and demands for evidence. This can become degrading because the sufferer is pushed into the role of witness to her own limitation. Cooking, painting and writing shift the evidence. They say: here is what was made. Here is the meal, the image, the page, the book, the press. Here is capacity, though not unlimited capacity. Here is life, though not easy life.

The distinction matters.

I do not want to be treated as incapable. I also do not want my visible capacities used to deny the severity of the condition. That is the narrow corridor many disabled people occupy. If we do nothing, we disappear into pity. If we do much, our disability is doubted. The task is to insist on both: I can make things, and I am in pain; I can think clearly, and I need to lie down; I can cook beautifully, and standing at the sink is nearly impossible; I can publish books, and carrying a box of books may be beyond me.

Both truths must be held.

The kitchen and the studio help hold them. They are places where limitation and capacity meet without cancelling each other. The body may dictate method, but it does not dictate meaning. A meal made in stages is still a meal. A painting made around pain is still a painting. A tea ceremony offered with unreliable hands is still an offering. A poem written in fragments is still a poem.

The fragment does not have to apologise.

This has become one of the central lessons of my life. Modern culture worships speed, visibility, productivity and seamless performance. Chronic pain destroys all four. It slows the body, hides the effort, makes productivity irregular and breaks performance into pieces. At first, this feels like failure. Later, if one is lucky or stubborn, it becomes another form of knowledge.

A life can be made through interrupted practices.

The meal can be started, paused, resumed. The painting can wait. The poem can hold one line until the next line comes. The book can grow across years. The publishing house can function through emails sent from bed. The legal argument can be built while the body rests. The tea can be prepared slowly. The day can be divided into tolerable units. The body may be unreliable, but the practices can remain faithful.

I have relied on practices more than moods.

Moods change. Hope rises and falls. Pain increases and retreats. Anger comes, then fatigue, then humour, then resignation, then energy, then pain again. Practices survive because they do not ask how one feels before they begin. They ask only for the next action. Fill the kettle. Open the file. Place the paper. Chop the onion. Rinse the brush. Check the proof. Write the sentence. Lie down. Begin again.

This is how a life continues.

If there is an advantage inside the disadvantage here, it lies in the precision of care. Bertolotti Syndrome has made care tangible. Care is not an abstract virtue. It is where the chair is placed. It is whether the meal can be cooked without collapse. It is whether the brush is within reach. It is whether a friend understands that tea may have to be made slowly. It is whether the book is shaped with enough attention to honour the person who needs it. It is whether the body is allowed to rest before it breaks.

In the kitchen, care becomes food.
In the studio, care becomes image.
On the page, care becomes language.
In publishing, care becomes a book.
In the body, care becomes survival.

These are not separate lives. They are one life, arranged around a spine that was never properly understood until too late.

The disadvantage is real. It has taken movement, money, ease, confidence, spontaneity and ordinary time. The advantage is more difficult to name without sounding sentimental. It is this: I have learned to make form under constraint. That is what cooking, painting, poetry, publishing, scholarship and pain have all required of me.

The body gave me constraint.

I answered with form.

15

The Flooded Cottage

A house is never only a house when the body is unreliable.

For a healthy person, unsuitable housing may be inconvenient, uncomfortable, irritating or expensive. For a person with Bertolotti Syndrome, it can become dangerous. The ordinary design of a home enters the body: steps, paths, flooring, drainage, cupboards, bathroom access, distance from the car, distance from the washing line, height of benches, weight of doors, the number of times one must bend, carry, mop, reach, lift or recover. Housing is not background. It is part of the medical condition.

From 2000 to 2026, I lived in Alice Springs. For much of that time, the town was the centre of my Australian life. I had work there, friends there, community there, history there. Alice Springs is not an easy place, but it is a place of force and memory. It had shaped me. I had written there, studied there, cooked there, painted there, founded Clear Mind Press there, built relationships there, and lived through many stages of the still-unnamed and then finally named condition.

From 2020, I rented a small cottage at the back of a property.

At first, it was simply a place to live. Later, it became one more site where my body and other people's indifference collided. By late 2025, when I finally received the Bertolotti Syndrome diagnosis, the cottage had already flooded seventeen times during periods of rain.

Alice Springs is in the desert. Rain is not constant. That can make flooding seem improbable to people who imagine the desert only as dryness. But when rain does come, it can come with force, and a badly drained property can become a trap. Three centimetres of muddy water through a home is not a minor inconvenience when the person living there has a disabling spinal condition.

Flooding is physical work.

It means mopping, lifting, moving, drying, bending, carrying, cleaning, sorting, assessing what has been damaged, trying to prevent further damage, and doing all of this while the body is already in pain. Muddy water does not wait politely while a person lies down. It enters. It spreads. It requires response. It turns the home into an emergency and the tenant into unpaid disaster labour.

Every flood cost me physically.

The landlords attempted repairs, but the repairs did not solve the problem. One of them described himself as a builder, yet even to me it was obvious that the drainage work was inadequate. The flooding continued. At one point, sandbags were placed across the path to my front door and then left there even during dry periods. For a person without mobility problems, sandbags across a path may be annoying. For me, they made access to the cottage difficult and painful.

A barrier to the front door is not a small thing.

The front door is the border between private life and the world. It is where groceries enter, friends arrive, parcels are delivered, emergency services would come if needed, and the person living there leaves for appointments, swimming, coffee, work or escape. When access to that door becomes physically difficult, the home begins to fail as a home.

This is where disability and housing meet. A house may be legally habitable in some general sense and still unsafe for a particular body. A repair may appear to have been attempted and still be ineffective. A landlord may think the problem is a maintenance inconvenience while the tenant experiences it as a direct threat to mobility, safety and health. The distance between those perspectives can become cruel.

Eventually, I asked the landlords to come to the cottage so that we could discuss the situation. I explained that the house was not safe for me, particularly in light of my diagnosis.

Their response was to tell me that I should leave.

Then, in front of me, they began discussing how much they might increase the rent for the next tenant.

That moment clarified the arrangement. My wellbeing was not central to them. My condition was not a matter requiring accommodation, care or urgency. It was an inconvenience. The problem, from their perspective, was not that a disabled tenant was living in a cottage that had flooded seventeen times. The problem was that I was still there.

I said I would leave as soon as I could find suitable alternative accommodation.

This was not simple. Finding housing in Alice Springs had become difficult. A few calls to local real estate agents quickly made clear that remaining there was not realistic. Rents were extremely high and the standard of available housing was poor. Suitable housing for someone with my condition was even harder to find. I did not need luxury. I needed safety, access, dryness, manageable layout, and a place where ordinary domestic life would not become a constant physical hazard.

Those requirements are modest. They are also not always easy to meet.

Because I ran a remote business, I could work from anywhere. That was one of the few advantages of the life I had built. Clear Mind Press did not require me to be in a particular street or town. My writing did not require a physical office. My legal scholarship did not depend on a local institution. The horizontal office was portable, provided there was an internet connection and enough physical stability to work.

This flexibility became escape.

I began looking elsewhere in Australia and quickly found a place in Queensland. Relocating became the obvious decision, although obvious does not mean easy. Moving house is physically demanding for almost anyone. For me, it was brutal. Packing a life requires bending, lifting, sorting, standing, carrying, twisting, decision-making, paperwork, phone calls, coordination, and the emotional labour of leaving a place where one has lived for decades.

By then, I was already depleted.

Repeated flooding had cost me. Cleaning and mopping had cost me. The diagnosis had not removed the pain. The medication episode had left its mark. The daily regime of swimming, rebounding, reformer work, rest and careful movement kept me functioning but did not give me reserves for crisis. A crisis consumes reserves a healthy person may not know she has. A person with chronic pain often has none to spare.

I informed the landlords that I would move as soon as the flooding on the route between Alice Springs and Queensland had eased. After that, the pressure increased. Although they knew about my diagnosis, their behaviour, as I experienced it, became passive-aggressive and seemed designed to force me out more quickly.

That is the phrasing I can use with care: as I experienced it.

A memoir is not a court judgment. I do not need to adjudicate every motive. I can record the effect. The effect was pressure. The effect was that my condition seemed to count for less than their desire to have the cottage empty. The effect was that a woman with a severe spinal condition was packing in pain under circumstances already made difficult by flooding, stress and the collapse of trust.

There is a particular loneliness in discovering that your vulnerability irritates people.

Not frightens them, not moves them, not calls them into responsibility, but irritates them. You become inconvenient. Your access needs are troublesome. Your safety concerns are delays. Your body's limits are obstacles to someone else's plan. In that moment, disability is revealed not only as a medical matter but as a social relation. The body hurts, but the social world decides whether that hurt is met with accommodation or impatience.

I have known both.

I have known friends who understand that I may need to lie down, leave early, avoid stairs, accept help or abandon a plan at short notice. I have known people who offer practical assistance without drama. I have known people who adapt the situation rather than expecting the body to adapt to an impossible situation. These people make life larger.

I have also known people who treat limitation as a nuisance.

The flooded cottage taught me again that chronic illness is never only internal. The spine is inside the body, but the consequences extend into buildings, tenancy, geography, weather, money, community and power. A landlord's indifference can worsen pain. A badly placed sandbag can increase risk. A poor rental market can force relocation. A remote business can make escape possible. A friend's help can become the difference between collapse and survival.

Housing is part of health.

This is an old truth, but chronic pain makes it immediate. A dry house, a safe path, a usable kitchen, a bathroom that does not require dangerous movement, a bedroom where rest is possible, a place to store medication or equipment, enough space for a reformer or rebounder, proximity to swimming, manageable maintenance: these are not lifestyle preferences. They are structural supports for a body under strain.

When those supports fail, the condition worsens.

I began packing. I packed books, papers, kitchen things, paintings, clothes, publishing materials, ordinary household objects and the accumulated remains of twenty-six years in Alice Springs. Packing is a confrontation with the material self. Every object asks whether it is worth carrying. For a person with pain, the question is literal. Is this worth lifting? Is this worth the space? Is this worth the movement? Is this worth the cost to the spine?

Books are especially difficult.

I am a writer and publisher. Books are my profession, my evidence, my tools, my companions and sometimes my burden. They are also heavy. A life made of books is a life made of boxes that the body may not be able to move. There is an irony in that which I did not find amusing at the time. The mind travels through books; the spine pays for their weight.

Packing forced selection. It also forced grief. Leaving a town after decades is not merely changing address. It is dismantling habits, routes, friendships, rooms, memories, routines, and a version of the self that belonged to that landscape. Alice Springs had been the place where I wrote, studied, loved, worked, struggled, built community and founded a press. It had also been the place of pain clinics, hospitalisations, flooding, diagnosis and the final exhaustion of trying to make a desert cottage safe.

A place can be both beloved and impossible.

That is difficult to explain to people who want decisions to be clean. Leaving Alice Springs was practical, but it was not emotionally simple. I did not leave only because of the landlords or the floods. I left because the body, the housing market, the medical possibilities and the future all pointed elsewhere. I needed warm water. I needed a safer home. I needed better access to medical systems. I needed a place where the physical environment did not constantly argue with my spine.

Queensland offered that possibility.

It also offered a symbolic movement: from desert to coast, from red dust to humidity, from a flooded cottage in an arid town to a subtropical place where swimming and warm water might become central to the day. I do not pretend that a new place cures a congenital spinal condition. I had learned too much to believe in geographical cures. But environment matters. Climate matters. Water matters. Housing matters. Access matters. A body in pain needs all the help the material world can give it.

The move was not a triumph. It was a necessity.

Still, necessity can contain direction. Bertolotti Syndrome had forced me many times to redesign life. The move to Queensland was one more redesign, larger than most. I took with me the horizontal office, the publishing house, the writer, the legal scholar, the cook, the painter, the walking stick, the fatigue, the pain, the habits of time management, the stubbornness, and the newly named spine.

I also took a clearer understanding of what I would no longer accept.

I would no longer accept a house that made the condition worse if I had any means of escape. I would no longer accept being treated as an inconvenience because my body required safety. I would no longer accept the idea that practical accommodations are favours. I would no longer accept the fiction that health begins and ends at the skin.

The body lives in systems.
The body lives in houses.
The body lives in weather.
The body lives in rent markets.
The body lives in the moral atmosphere created by other people.

The flooded cottage was part of my Bertolotti story because it showed what happens when a vulnerable body meets an unsafe environment and indifferent power. It was not separate from the medical condition. It was the condition expressed through housing.

The spine had been malformed from birth. The cottage had been unsafe by design or neglect. The first was anatomy. The second was avoidable.

That distinction matters.

I cannot change the vertebra I was born with. Other people can change how they respond to a person living with its consequences. They can listen. They can repair properly. They can remove barriers. They can avoid making safety a negotiation. They can refrain from treating disability as an inconvenience. They can understand that chronic pain already takes enough without the built environment adding its own demands.

Leaving Alice Springs was one of the hardest acts of practical self-protection I have undertaken. It required the same discipline the whole condition had required: assess reality, stop hoping the wrong thing will improve, use the available window, move before the body is pushed beyond recovery, and accept that a life sometimes has to be rebuilt from the horizontal.

By the time I left, I was exhausted.

But I was leaving.

16

Warm Water

Queensland did not cure me. It gave me better conditions.

That distinction matters. I had lived too long with pain to believe in geographical salvation. I knew that a congenital spinal condition does not disappear because the air is warmer, the sea is closer, the fruit is brighter, or the garden more generous. The spine travels with the person. It arrives in the new house, lies down in the new room, wakes in the new bed, and begins its daily negotiations as before.

Yet place matters.

The body does not live in abstraction. It lives in temperature, light, humidity, paths, chairs, floors, kitchens, bathrooms, gardens, distances and weather. It lives in the space between the bed and the kettle, the car and the front door, the pool and the change room, the chair and the table, the garden and the kitchen. A body in pain is exquisitely sensitive to its environment because the environment is never neutral. It either helps or hinders. It either softens the day or makes every movement more expensive.

Queensland softened the day.

After the harshness of Central Australia, the coast felt almost excessive. Sun, sea, warm air, wet green growth, birds, fruit, flowers, salt, cloud, rain, and that great open wash of light that belongs to the edge of the ocean. The place did not have the fierce, ancient austerity of Alice Springs. It had abundance. It was leafy, humid, alive, almost indecently fertile. Things grew because that is what things did there. A branch cut back would return. Herbs sprang forward. Fruit appeared. Vines moved. The garden did not stand there like an image. It worked.

I had moved from a flooded cottage in the desert to a place where water belonged.

That changed something in me before it changed anything in my body. The sea gave scale. The sky widened differently. The air carried moisture rather than dust. The sun had a softer authority. Even the mornings seemed to arrive with food in them: pawpaw, herbs, greens, citrus, tomatoes, whatever could be found, gathered, traded, bought locally or taken from the garden before the day grew too warm.

Fresh produce became part of the new life almost immediately. There is a particular pleasure in food that still seems attached to the soil. Fruit with sun in it. Greens that have not travelled halfway across the continent. Herbs cut because they are there. A garden where one can forage changes the relationship between cooking and place. The meal begins before the kitchen. It begins with walking slowly through green abundance, noticing what is ready, what has ripened, what can be used, what should be left another day.

For me, that kind of foraging had to be modest. The body still set limits. I could not stroll indefinitely, bend freely, carry heavily or stand too long at the bench afterwards. But even a small act of gathering gave the day a different quality. A few herbs. A lemon. Leaves for a salad. Something unexpected from the garden. These are small things, but chronic pain teaches respect for small things. The large freedoms may be gone; the small freedoms acquire force.

The kitchen changed with the garden.

Cooking in Queensland became brighter, fresher and more immediate. Less heavy, more colour. Less endurance, more arrangement. A meal could be built around what the place offered: fruit, vegetables, herbs, sea air, heat, shade, and the kind of appetite that belongs near water. The body still objected to standing at the sink. The stove still required negotiation. The washing up remained the enemy. But the ingredients themselves brought energy.

A sliced tomato can be a declaration of place. So can a handful of basil, a bowl of fruit, a simple meal eaten in warm light. Pain does not erase such things. Sometimes it makes them more necessary.

I began to understand Queensland as a form of environmental assistance. No doctor prescribed it. No allied health professional wrote it into a plan. Yet the sun, water, garden and local produce became part of the architecture of living with Bertolotti Syndrome. The condition remained. The setting became kinder.

Warm water helped most.

Swimming had already become central to my health regime, but Queensland made it feel less like a survival task and more like a natural extension of the day. The water supported the body. It allowed movement without the same brutality of gravity. It gave me a temporary version of myself that could move with less fear. In water, I am still careful, but I am less trapped. The body is not weightless, but it is less accused.

The sea itself offered another form of therapy, although I hesitate to use that word because it has been applied too often to things that did not help. The sea did not treat Bertolotti Syndrome. It did not diagnose, inject, operate or prescribe. It gave rhythm, horizon and sensory relief. It reminded me that the body is part of the natural world, not merely a defective mechanism moving between appointments. Salt air, sun on the skin, the sound of water, a line of pelicans, the brightness of a Queensland morning: these do not cure pain, but they alter its company.

Pain in a beautiful place is still pain. It is also pain with a view.

That may sound trivial. It is not. The surroundings of suffering matter. A flooded cottage, sandbags across the door and muddy water through the house create one kind of pain-world. A warm coast, fresh produce, a generous garden and a friend who understands create another. The spine may be the same. The life around it is altered.

The friendship mattered as much as the climate.

A super nice friendship is not a small thing at this stage of life. I use the phrase deliberately because it resists solemnity. There are friendships that are formally admirable, and there are friendships that make daily life lighter. This was the second kind. Practical, funny, generous, undramatic. The kind of friendship where the other person does not need a lecture on disability to understand that a chair matters, that carrying things matters, that a visit may need to be short, that lying down is not an insult to the conversation.

Pain tests friendship because it removes ease. It asks whether the other person can tolerate adjustment. Some people cannot. They need spontaneity, long outings, conventional posture, cheerful endurance and the illusion that everyone present is operating under similar physical conditions. Others adapt immediately. They make room. They do not make a performance of making room. They simply include the body as it is.

This friendship gave me that.

It gave me companionship without constant explanation. It gave me humour. It gave me practical help when practical help mattered. It gave me the sense that the move had not only removed me from an unsafe situation but delivered me into a more generous human arrangement. After years of forcing myself through systems, appointments, tenancy stress, flooding and the ordinary loneliness of pain, that generosity had a physical effect. The nervous system notices safety.

The choir was another unexpected opening.

Singing in a choir is a strange gift for someone whose body has become so restricted. It is social, disciplined and embodied without requiring the same sort of movement that walking, standing or dancing demand. It uses breath, listening, timing, attention and the willingness to belong to a sound larger than one's own voice. A choir is a community organised through vibration. Each person brings a line, but no one carries the whole.

That suited me.

Pain can make a person solitary even when she does not wish to be. Social life becomes difficult because ordinary gatherings are arranged around bodies that can sit, stand, walk, linger and recover easily. A choir gives structure. There is a time to arrive, a place to sit or stand as one can, music to follow, other voices to lean into, and a shared purpose that is neither medical nor domestic nor professional. It is not about the back. It is not about diagnosis. It is not about publishing, law or survival. It is about sound.

That is a relief.

The voice comes from the body, of course. There is no escape from embodiment. But singing relates to the body differently from pain. Pain contracts attention. Singing expands it. Pain isolates sensation. Singing blends it with breath and other voices. Pain says: here, here, here, this point, this joint, this muscle, this nerve. Singing says: listen outward; enter the chord; hold your note; breathe with others.

It reminded me of dance, but without the same physical demand. It gave form to breath. It gave company to discipline.

Art also returned more strongly.

Queensland had light for painting. Different light from the desert. Less severe, more humid, more reflective, more green. The colour palette shifted because the place insisted on it. After the red earth and hard lines of Central Australia, the coast offered softness, saturation, leaf shadow, water, fruit, flowers and the everyday drama of things growing too well. The visual world became fuller.

That mattered to the painter in me.

Art had always been one way of looking carefully. In Queensland, looking became less forensic and more sensual. The silhouettes had been evidence: look at the body, look at the asymmetry, look at what was missed. The new work could still carry pain, but it did not have to prove it. There was room for colour, plants, water, faces, domestic objects, the garden, the sea, the strangeness of a body still hurting in a place so alive.

This was important because illness can turn art into testimony. Testimony matters, but art needs more than testimony. It needs play, risk, composition, surprise and pleasure. Queensland gave some of that back. The body remained limited, but the visual field expanded. I could look outwards again.

The garden helped. A garden is a living studio. It makes compositions without permission: leaves against sky, fruit against shadow, a path half covered, a bowl of gathered produce, the disorder of growth, the sudden elegance of a flower placed where no human would have placed it. A painter can learn from a garden because a garden understands arrangement without rigidity.

A cook can learn from it too.

There is a direct line between garden, kitchen and table. Foraging turns cooking into a conversation with place. A recipe may begin with an ingredient, but a garden begins with availability. What is ripe? What is abundant? What is about to spoil? What can be cut without damaging the plant? What needs using today? These questions are practical and ecological. They also suit a life of constraint because they begin from what is actually available, rather than from an ideal plan imposed from elsewhere.

That, in a sense, is the whole method of living with Bertolotti Syndrome.

Begin from what is actually available.
Not the body one wishes for.
Not the day one planned.
Not the energy one had ten years ago.
Not the social expectation.
Not the doctor's generic advice.
The actual available body.
The actual available time.
The actual available garden.
The actual available light.

Then make something.

Queensland did not remove the need for calculation. I still had to manage standing, sitting, walking, fatigue, cooking, swimming, social life and work. I still had to lie down. I still had pain. I still had the walking stick. I still had to protect the day from collapse. The difference was that the calculations took place inside a more generous environment. The world around me had become less adversarial.

That allowed more life to enter.

There were mornings when the sun itself seemed to tell me to begin again. There were days when the sea made the body's misery less claustrophobic. There were meals that tasted of the garden. There were choir rehearsals where breath and sound carried me beyond the private weather of pain. There were conversations with a friend that did not require translation. There were colours I wanted to paint. There were manuscripts to edit, books to design, legal thoughts to finish, and food to make from whatever the garden had offered.

This is the vibrant part of the story, but it should not be mistaken for a happy ending.

A happy ending would require the pain to end. It has not ended. A happy ending would require the decades to be restored. They cannot be restored. A happy ending would require the money, strength, opportunities and confidence to come back. They will not.

Queensland offered something more modest and therefore more believable. It offered better terms.

Better terms are not nothing.

After a lifetime of being forced to adapt to systems, practitioners, climates, houses and explanations that did not fit, I had found a place that adapted itself more easily to the body I actually had. Warm water. Sun. Sea. Fresh produce. A garden generous enough to forage. A friendship that made space without fuss. A choir. More art. More colour. A life still constrained, but less starved.

The advantage in the disadvantage became easier to see there.

In Central Australia, the body had often been tested by hardness: distance, heat, dust, housing, isolation, flooded rooms, sandbags and medical scarcity. In Queensland, the body encountered softness without weakness. The softness of water, humidity, fruit, leaves, friendship, song and colour. Softness can be strong. It can hold a person together in ways discipline alone cannot.

I had lived for decades on discipline.

Now I could add abundance.

Not unlimited abundance. Not careless abundance. I remain a person who measures the day. But abundance of another kind: sensory, social, culinary, aesthetic. A bowl of fruit. A handful of herbs. Sea light. A good friend. A choir chord. A painting table. A swim. A meal. A manuscript. A morning that does not begin with the feeling that the environment itself is against me.

These things matter because a painful life needs more than management. It needs reasons.

Management keeps the body functioning. Reasons keep the person alive inside the management. Queensland gave me reasons in bright, ordinary forms. It gave me reasons to cook, to sing, to paint, to swim, to step into the garden, to notice the sky, to make a meal, to answer a friend, to keep the press going, to let the day contain more than defence.

The body remained tyrannical.

It was no longer the only government.

17

Every Disadvantage

The Dutch saying is usually given as *elk nadeel heeft zijn voordeel*: every disadvantage has its advantage.

It is not a soft saying. That is why I like it. It does not pretend that the disadvantage is secretly good. It does not say that suffering is noble, or that pain improves the soul, or that everything happens for a reason. It simply says that the disadvantage may contain an advantage. The advantage has to be found, made, forced, recognised or extracted. It does not arrive as compensation. It is not owed to us.

Bertolotti Syndrome has been the great disadvantage of my life.

It has cost me movement, money, sleep, confidence, spontaneity, relationships, work, ease, and decades of medical clarity. It has cost me approximately $1.2 million in doctors, therapists, medications, shoes, equipment, treatment experiments, exercise regimes, alternative health interventions, lost opportunities and the slow financial leakage of trying to solve a problem without knowing what it was. It has cost me the freedom to stand at a sink, sit in a café without calculation, walk without a stick, cook without strategy, travel without fear, or accept an invitation without first assessing the chair, the distance and the exit route.

It has cost too much to romanticise.

The advantage was never the pain. I want that stated clearly. Pain itself did not make me better, wiser, kinder or more interesting. Pain made many things harder. It made some things impossible. It made me frightened, impatient, exhausted and sometimes furious. It made me dependent in ways I disliked. It made me vulnerable to bad theories and bad practitioners. It sent me into rooms where I should not have had to go and kept me in systems that should have looked properly the first time.

The advantage was what I had to build because the pain would not leave.

I had to build method. I had to build discipline. I had to build a way of working from the horizontal. I had to build a life in fragments and then learn not to despise the fragments. I had to build a kitchen practice, a writing practice, an art practice, a publishing practice and a scholarly practice around a body that gave me unreliable access to ordinary time. I had to decide what mattered because the body would not allow me to do everything.

That is a hard teacher.

A healthy person may have the luxury of vagueness. I do not. Vague plans collapse quickly when the body is expensive to move. I need to know what the task is, where the object is, how long I can stand, whether I can sit, whether I can lie down afterwards, whether the action is worth the cost, whether the day has enough reserve left for one more thing. This has made me exacting. It has made me impatient with pointless complexity, bad systems, sloppy thinking and sentimental language that does not survive contact with the facts.

That exactness has served my work.

It served the writer who changed languages. It served the poet working inside the discipline of form. It served the painter learning to look properly. It served the cook who knows that a meal is built through sequence, timing and care. It served the publisher who understands that a book needs a spine, structure, attention and finish. It served the legal scholar trying to understand what justice requires when systems fail to see the whole field.

The body trained the mind by refusing ease.

This is not a recommendation. I would not prescribe Bertolotti Syndrome to anyone as a route to discipline. There are easier ways to learn time management. There are kinder ways to develop insight. If I could have been diagnosed properly at twenty-one, or thirty, or forty, I would have taken that life. I would have preferred informed treatment to character formation. I would have preferred a functioning spine to philosophical clarity. I would have preferred money spent on houses, travel, family, art, books and pleasure rather than on decades of wrong answers.

Still, this is the life I have.

The question, then, is not whether the disadvantage should have happened. It should not have happened in the way it did. The question is what can be made now, with the body, knowledge, anger, humour, discipline and time that remain.

For many years, I believed the problem was that I had not found the right cure. That belief kept me searching. It also kept me vulnerable. After diagnosis, the search changed. I stopped asking every new method to save me. I began asking a more practical question: what helps me remain myself?

That question is better.

Swimming helps. Warm water helps. Rest helps. The Pilates reformer helps. The rebounder helps. A chair that does not punish me helps. A garden helps. A friend who understands helps. Good food helps. A publishing problem that absorbs the mind helps. Art helps. A choir helps. Legal thinking helps. Poetry helps. A room arranged around reality helps. A diagnosis helps, even when it comes late.

Recognition helps.

For most of my life, the real struggle was not only pain. It was the gap between the pain I felt and the explanations I was given. That gap damaged me. It produced self-doubt, anxiety, wasted labour and a long procession of treatments aimed at the wrong thing. When the pain clinic doctor drew the structure and wrote "Bertolotti Syndrome", she did not heal my back. She healed part of the fracture between bodily truth and social reality.

There is justice in being believed by someone who knows what she is looking at.

That is why this book is also about systems. A patient can be brave, disciplined, informed and persistent, and still be harmed by a system that lacks the right frame. A doctor can be kind and still miss the thing that matters. A scan can show anatomy and still fail to produce diagnosis. A legal system can process a person and still miss the actual harm. A housing arrangement can be technically ordinary and still be unsafe for a disabled body. A society can praise productivity while refusing to see what that productivity costs.

The body is never only private.

It lives in medicine, housing, work, money, friendship, climate, gender, age, language, and law. My spine may be congenital, but my suffering was shaped by many human arrangements: what doctors knew, what they dismissed, what images were interpreted to mean, what treatments were offered, what rent I could afford, what houses were available, what friends understood, what work could be done lying down, what technologies allowed remote publishing, what swimming pools and gardens and warm climates made possible.

A disadvantage is rarely solitary. It sits inside systems.

So does an advantage.

The advantage in my life came partly from temperament. I am stubborn. I like making things. I do not give up easily. I can work intensely in small windows. I can live in ideas. I can turn a sentence over until it becomes clean. I can build a book. I can cook something good from what is available. I can look at a problem until its structure begins to show. These qualities helped me survive.

But temperament is not enough. I also needed tools, books, water, friends, internet, language, education, a laptop, a bed, a garden, and eventually a diagnosis. No one survives pain by character alone. That is another romantic lie.

What I have survived, I have survived through arrangements.

The fifteen-minute life is an arrangement. Sovereign Health is an arrangement. Clear Mind Press is an arrangement. The horizontal office is an arrangement. The kitchen in stages is an arrangement. The Queensland garden is an arrangement. The choir is an arrangement. Friendship is an arrangement of care. A book is an arrangement of attention.

Perhaps this is the deeper lesson. A life does not have to be large in movement to be large in arrangement. It can be built carefully, from fragments, if the fragments are given form.

When I look back now, I see the child stumbling in the Netherlands. I see her mother becoming irritated because the walk to the shops has slowed down. I see the skeleton poster, the marbles picked up with toes, the red linen *Grimm's Fairy Tales* balanced on the head. I see the dancer with one impossible side. I see the young mother in Ghent, carrying babies and wearing the wrong shoe. I see the woman in Tokyo, trusting Wakui's hands, sitting in sulphur water, then throwing away the drawing. I see the Amsterdam years of wedges, hammers and wine. I see New South Wales, Nimbin, Sarno, Buddhism and the monastery. I see Alice Springs, hospital rooms, pain clinics, flooding, sandbags and packing boxes. I see the doctor drawing my spine. I see Queensland, warm water, fresh produce, art, friendship and song.

All of these women are me.

The diagnosis made them continuous. The book gives them sequence. Without the diagnosis, the story was scattered into episodes. With the diagnosis, it became legible. That is another advantage, though a late one. I can now tell the story correctly. I can say that the body was speaking from the beginning. I can say that competence hid suffering. I can say that the pain was not imaginary. I can say that the misdiagnosis was not a personal failure. I can say that an undiagnosed congenital spinal condition shaped the way I became a writer, poet, painter, cook, publisher and legal scholar.

It did not create those lives. It altered their practice.

I wrote lying down. I cooked in stages. I painted around pain. I published from bed. I studied law through fragments. I organised my days according to what the body would permit. I became precise because imprecision hurt. I became efficient because waste had consequences. I became suspicious of narrow systems because my own life had been narrowed by them. I became attentive because inattention had cost me decades.

There is the advantage.

It is not consolation. It is not moral redemption. It is a usable remainder.

The disadvantage is that my life has been physically smaller than it might have been. The advantage is that I learned to make the remaining space dense. Dense with books, food, paintings, poems, arguments, friendships, gardens, publishing projects, swims, songs, research, and the stubborn refusal to become only a patient.

I do not know what comes next medically. Perhaps another doctor will listen. Perhaps some intervention remains possible. Perhaps not. I have learned not to place too much of my life in the hands of a future appointment. Hope is useful only when it does not empty the present.

The present is where I still have work to do.

There are books to publish. There are meals to prepare. There are poems to shape. There are paintings to finish. There are friends to see, though not for too long in the wrong chair. There is a choir to attend. There is water to enter. There is fruit in the garden. There are manuscripts waiting. There are legal questions that still matter. There is a body that will have to lie down again soon.

This is not the life I would have chosen.

It is, however, a life.

That may sound modest, but modest claims are sometimes the most exact. I have lived with a condition that was missed for nearly half a century. I have paid for that omission in almost every currency a life contains. Yet the same life also produced work, art, food, scholarship, books, friendship and a method of living that belongs to me.

Every disadvantage has its advantage.

The saying does not erase the disadvantage. It asks what can still be done with it.

My answer is this book.

18

For Anyone Still Searching

This book began with one woman's spine, but it should not end there.

There are many people living with pain that has not been properly named. Some of them are young. Some are old. Some have been told their scans are normal. Some have been told the findings on their scans are incidental. Some have been told the problem is muscular, postural, psychological, stress-related, age-related, weight-related, hormonal, emotional, ordinary or mysterious. Some have been told to try another round of physiotherapy, another medication, another mindfulness course, another exercise regime, another practitioner, another explanation that sounds plausible enough to postpone the right question.

Some of them have Bertolotti Syndrome and do not yet know it.

This book cannot diagnose anyone. It is not a substitute for medical care. A person with persistent back pain should seek proper medical advice, and any treatment decision has to be made with an appropriately qualified clinician. But there is a difference between self-diagnosis and informed questioning. A patient is allowed to ask better questions. A patient is allowed to say: this pain began young; this pain keeps returning; this pain does not behave like ordinary backache; this pain is made worse by standing, sitting, walking, lifting, bending or twisting; this pain settles when I rest; this pain has not been explained. Could this be Bertolotti Syndrome?

That question may change the path.

It may not. Many back problems are not Bertolotti Syndrome. Many people have lumbosacral transitional vertebrae without symptoms. Many people have more than one condition, and the spine is a complex structure in which discs, joints, nerves, muscles, ligaments, fascia, pelvis and hips may all contribute to pain. The point is not to make Bertolotti Syndrome the explanation for every stubborn backache. The point is to ensure that it is not missed when the pattern fits.

Being missed is not a neutral event.

A missed diagnosis consumes time. It consumes money. It consumes trust. It sends the patient into treatments that may be irrelevant, ineffective or harmful. It may convert structural pain into psychological suspicion. It may encourage people to push through when rest would be wiser. It may lead to operations directed at the wrong structure. It may leave a young person living through the most active decades of life with a body that is not understood by the very people meant to help.

That was my story. It should not have to be yours.

If you are reading this because you are in pain, I want to say this plainly: severe pain that has not yet been properly explained is not evidence that you are unreliable. It is evidence that the explanation has not yet been adequate. There may be psychological consequences. There may be fear, depression, anger, trauma, guarding, central sensitisation, fatigue and despair. All of these may need care. But psychological consequences do not automatically mean psychological cause.

Hold that distinction carefully.

It took me too long to hold it. For years, I tried to persuade my brain to stop producing pain. I journalled, meditated, analysed, studied, sat in monasteries, talked to my brain, searched my past and tried to become more spiritually and psychologically correct. Some of that work helped me live with pain. None of it changed the abnormal bony structure at the base of my spine. Some methods soothe the nervous system. Some give attention back to the body. Some reduce fear. Those things have value. They become dangerous when they tell a person to stop looking for the structural cause that is actually there.

A malformed spine cannot be journalled into normal anatomy.

That sentence may sound obvious, but many people in pain need permission to say it. The modern world likes explanations that turn suffering into a matter of attitude, trauma, belief, lifestyle or personal growth. Some suffering does involve those things. Some suffering also involves bone. A just approach to pain must leave room for both without collapsing one into the other.

The body deserves to be believed, but it also deserves to be investigated properly. Belief alone is not enough. A kind doctor who does not know what to look for may still miss the diagnosis. A confident practitioner may still be confidently wrong. A scan may be done but interpreted through an inadequate frame. A transitional vertebra may be mentioned and then dismissed as incidental, even when it deserves further clinical attention. The patient may therefore need both respect and specificity.

Respect says: I believe that your pain is real.

Specificity asks: what structure is causing it?

For Bertolotti Syndrome, that specificity matters. The question is not simply whether an anatomical variant exists. The question is whether the transitional segment is clinically significant. That requires proper imaging, careful correlation with symptoms, clinical reasoning and, in some cases, diagnostic injections. The diagnostic injection is important because it can help determine whether the suspected structure is actually generating the pain. Without that step, treatment may proceed on assumption, and assumption has already ruined too many lives.

Doctors need to know this. Patients need to know this too.

A patient should not have to educate her doctor, but sometimes she must. That is one of the practical indignities of an under-recognised condition. The patient arrives in pain, often exhausted, and is then required to become a researcher, advocate, file manager and educator. It is unfair. It is also sometimes necessary. If your doctor does not know about Bertolotti Syndrome, that does not mean the condition is unimportant. It may mean only that medical training has not given the condition sufficient attention.

Bring information. Ask questions. Keep copies of scans and reports. Ask whether the lumbosacral junction has been properly assessed. Ask whether the radiologist has specifically commented on transitional anatomy. Ask whether further imaging is needed. Ask whether a diagnostic injection is appropriate. Ask whether the clinician treating you has experience with Bertolotti Syndrome. Ask what else could explain the symptoms. Ask what is known, what is uncertain, and what is being assumed.

A good doctor should welcome informed questions.

A poor one may become irritated.

I do not say this to make patients distrust every doctor. Distrust can become exhausting in its own right. Medicine contains many intelligent, humane and careful people. My diagnosis arrived because one doctor knew what she was looking at and took the time to draw it. That moment changed my life, even though it came late. The lesson is not that medicine is useless. The lesson is that medicine must remain curious.

Curiosity is a clinical virtue.

It is also a human one. Family and friends need it as well. A person with chronic pain may appear inconsistent: able to do something one day and unable the next; articulate in conversation but physically close to collapse; productive in work but unable to stand at the sink; cheerful at lunch but in bed afterwards; capable of writing a book but unable to carry the box the books arrive in. This inconsistency is not deceit. It is the ordinary variability of a body under strain.

Competence hides pain.
Good clothes hide pain.
Clear speech hides pain.
Humour hides pain.
Productivity hides pain.
A made meal hides pain.
A published book hides pain.

Do not make the mistake of thinking that because a person can still do something, the condition cannot be severe. Partial ability is one of the most misunderstood features of chronic illness. It allows life to continue, but it also makes suffering less visible. Many people with Bertolotti Syndrome and other chronic pain conditions live in this gap. They are too functional to be believed fully and too impaired to live freely.

The practical kindnesses matter.

A good chair matters. A place to lie down matters. A shorter visit matters. Help carrying things matters. A meal matters. A lift matters. Not taking cancellation personally matters. Not offering a theory matters. Not telling the person to think positively matters. Asking what would make the visit possible matters. Believing that pain can be severe even when the person is still clever, funny and productive matters.

The medical system often thinks in large interventions. Surgery, medication, injections, imaging, rehabilitation. Those may be necessary. But daily life is often sustained by small accommodations. The object placed within reach. The task divided. The heavy thing carried by someone else. The path kept clear. The house kept dry. The visit shortened. The work done remotely. The couch made available. These are not luxuries. They are part of the architecture of functioning.

I learned this through necessity. I learned to arrange my life around small windows of capacity. Fifteen minutes at the sink. Fifteen minutes at the stove. Fifteen minutes standing, then lying down. A paragraph, a rest, another paragraph. A swim, a recovery, an email. A meal made in stages. A publishing house run from the bed. A legal argument built through fragments. A poem held until the next line arrived.

The fragment became a unit of life.

If you are living in fragments, do not despise them. A fragment is not a failed whole. It is the form available today. A life can be built from fragments if they are treated with respect. The danger is to compare every day with the body you once had, the body other people have, or the body you were told you should have if only you tried harder. That comparison can become another form of injury.

Begin with the actual body. Begin with the actual hour. Begin with the actual energy. Begin with what is within reach.

Then make something.

It may be a meal, a phone call, a paragraph, a shower, an appointment, a stretch, a swim, a short walk, a message to a doctor, a question written down for the next consultation, a painting, a poem, a rest before collapse. The act may seem small from the outside. It may be large from within the body that performs it. The scale of an action should be measured by the cost to the person doing it, not by the casual judgement of those who do not have to pay.

I have paid dearly for not knowing what was wrong with my body. I have paid in money, time, opportunities, trust and ordinary ease. Yet I have also learned that a person can remain intellectually and creatively alive inside a severely restricted body. That is not a consolation prize. It is a form of survival.

Survival deserves precision.

It is not always heroic. Much of it is dull. It is forms, appointments, devices, waiting lists, laundry, meals, rest, pain, sleep, small plans, cancelled outings, medical reports, and the quiet work of beginning again after yet another disappointment. But inside that dullness, there can still be dignity. Dignity does not require triumph. It requires being treated, and treating oneself, as a whole person.

That is what I want for anyone still searching.

I want you to be treated as a whole person. Not a spine. Not an anxious patient. Not a difficult case. Not a pain identity. Not a scan. Not an incidental finding. Not a psychological puzzle. Not a set of muscles. Not a nuisance. A person, with a body, a history, work, relationships, fears, capacities, intelligence, humour, anger and a future that deserves not to be wasted by the wrong explanation.

Keep asking the right questions.

Do it calmly when you can. Do it fiercely when you must. Take someone with you if you need support. Write down the history. Keep the images. Read enough to ask intelligently, but do not let research consume the life you are trying to protect. Find others with the condition if that helps. Patient communities can contain practical knowledge that official pathways have been slow to gather. Use them carefully, but do not dismiss them. Many of us found recognition first through other patients.

Most of all, do not let anyone convert your unresolved pain into a defect of character.

The body may be difficult. The search may be long. The answer may be partial. The treatment may be uncertain. Still, you are entitled to proper attention. You are entitled to ask whether the person looking at your spine knows what to look for. You are entitled to rest. You are entitled to adapt. You are entitled to make a life that does not look conventional but remains yours.

I lost almost fifty years to an unnamed condition.

I cannot get those years back. But I can write this, and perhaps that is one form of return: to take the long, expensive, humiliating search and turn it into a signpost for someone else. If even one person asks the right question earlier because of this book, the story has done work beyond my own life.

That matters.

A book cannot hold up a spine.

It can hold open a door.

19

Note to Those Living with Chronic Pain

I have written this book for people living with Bertolotti Syndrome, and also for everyone who lives with chronic pain, chronic illness, fatigue, disability or a body that has become difficult to trust.

I want this story to offer recognition. Chronic illness can make a person feel as if life has become smaller, slower and less visible to others. Pain can remove ease from ordinary things: standing at a sink, sitting through a meal, carrying shopping, keeping appointments, working, travelling, making plans, seeing friends, or simply beginning the day. It can also make a person feel misread. People may see competence and assume wellness. They may see productivity and assume capacity. They may see a smile, a book, a meal, a painting, a job, or a conversation and miss the cost behind it.

My hope is that this book shows another possibility. A restricted body does not have to mean a diminished life. Life may have to be redesigned. Time may have to be broken into smaller units. Work may have to be done lying down. Friendship may need clearer boundaries. Creativity may need different methods. Rest may have to become part of the structure of the day rather than an apology for what cannot be done. Yet within those altered conditions, a life can still contain thought, humour, beauty, usefulness, friendship, art, food, scholarship, work and meaning.

I do not write this from a place of cure. I write from adaptation. I still live with pain. I still have to measure my day carefully. I still need to lie down. I still have to decide which tasks are worth the physical cost. This book therefore offers no fantasy that illness can be overcome by attitude. It offers something more practical: the possibility of remaining oneself under constraint.

If you are living with chronic pain or chronic illness, I hope this book encourages you to believe your own body, protect your energy, ask better questions, seek proper care, and refuse shame. I hope it helps you see that small windows of capacity still count. A paragraph, a meal, a swim, a phone call, a drawing, a rest, a question written down for the doctor, a short visit with a friend: these are not failed versions of a larger life. They are the life available today, and they deserve respect.

Pain can take a great deal. It should not be allowed to take the whole self.

20

Bertolotti Curve

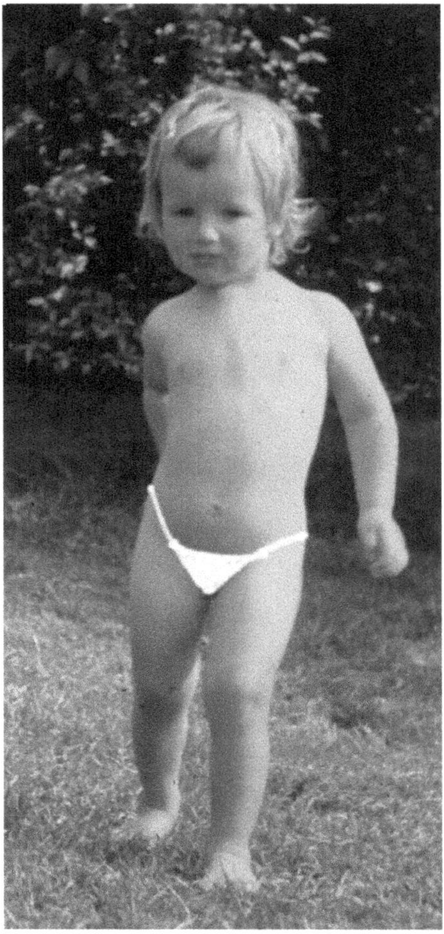

ABOUT THIS BOOK

For nearly fifty years, Suzanne Visser lived with severe lower back pain without knowing its cause. Doctors, specialists, therapists and alternative practitioners offered explanations: posture, childbirth, muscle tension, anxiety, wear and tear, repressed emotion, even the joints in her face. None of them named the condition she had been born with: Bertolotti Syndrome.

By the time the diagnosis finally arrived, the cost of not knowing had been immense — physically, emotionally and financially. Suzanne estimates that approximately $1.2 million had been spent, lost or diverted through decades of misdiagnosis, treatments, equipment, medication, special shoes, lost opportunities and the ordinary economic leakage of chronic pain.

Yet this is not only a story about illness. It is the story of a life built under constraint: a writer who changed languages, a poet, painter, cook, publisher and legal scholar who learned to work in fragments, often lying down, often in pain, and often within windows of only fifteen minutes. Through motherhood, migration, Japan, Australia, law, publishing, art, cooking, friendship and late diagnosis, Suzanne's story asks what can still be made when the body will not co-operate.

The Million-Dollar Misdiagnosis: Living, Writing and Creating with Bertolotti Syndrome is a memoir about chronic pain, medical dismissal, time, creativity and survival. It offers recognition to those still searching for a name for their pain, and a clear-eyed account of how a restricted body can still contain an intellectually and creatively expansive life.

Suzanne H Visser is a Dutch-born Australian writer, poet, painter, publisher and legal scholar. She began her writing career in the Netherlands before later making Australia her home. Her work has crossed languages, countries and genres, including fiction, poetry, essays, legal scholarship and non-fiction.

Suzanne is the founder and director of Clear Mind Press, an independent Australian publishing house. Through the press, she publishes books that are intellectually serious, socially engaged and often difficult to place within conventional commercial categories. Her own writing includes literary fiction, poetry, books on justice, creativity, ageing, and the human search for meaning.

She completed her doctoral work in law on the concept of Sustainable Justice, exploring how legal systems might respond more adequately to complexity, long-term consequences, ecological responsibility and human wellbeing. Her legal scholarship is shaped by a lifelong concern with systems that fail to see what is directly in front of them.

Suzanne was diagnosed with Bertolotti Syndrome after nearly five decades of chronic lower back pain and repeated misdiagnosis across several countries. Much of her work is now done lying down, in carefully managed periods of concentration. Rather than allowing severe physical constraint to define the limits of her life, she has continued to write, publish, paint, cook, study, sing, swim and build creative structures around the body she has.

After many years in Alice Springs, Suzanne now lives in Queensland, where warm water, a generous garden, fresh produce, friendship, choir singing and art form part of her continuing practice of living with pain without surrendering the whole self to it.

Available from Clear Mind Press

Justice That Can Last

Bertolotti Syndrome: An Underdiagnosed Cause of Back Pain

Find Your iKiGAi

The Great Kitschification: Why AI Will Never Be Good at Art

The Mankeeper

Hundred Fifty Five Sonnets

Life Force

Never Retire: An Exploration of Old Age

Cash!

Marks on Paper: Essays on Drawing, Seeing and Looking

The Elephant's Tooth: Crime in Rural Australia

The Elephant's Tooth: Crime in Alice Springs

The Fish Murders

Earlier work

I, Unborn, Undying: A Search for the Self

De pracht van het dagelijks leven

De Vismoorden

De Verdwijning

Terra Nostra

Een man met mooie benen

De Vismoorden was later published in German as *Das Japanische Rätsel,* in French as *Les Meurtres au Poisson,* in Spanish as *Sushi,* and in English as *The Fish Murders.*

https://www.clearmindpress.com/

The Million Dollar Misdiagnosis: Living, Writing and Creating with Bertolotti Syndrome

Published by Clear Mind Press, 2026, in Craignish QLD, Australia

ISBN Print: 978-1-7647914-2-7

EISBN Ebook: 978-1-7647914-3-4

Typeset: Clear Mind Press

Cover design: Clear Mind Press

Portrait of the author: Hazel Blake

Photo of Suzanne as a child: Henk Visser.

https://www.clearmindpress.com

Notes